Vaccination

Recent Titles in Contemporary Debates

VACCINATION

Examining the Facts

Lisa Rosner

Contemporary Debates

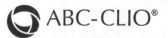
ABC-CLIO®

An Imprint of ABC-CLIO, LLC
Santa Barbara, California • Denver, Colorado

Library of Congress Control Number: 2022012544

ISBN: 978-1-4408-7760-5 (print)
      978-1-4408-7761-2 (ebook)

26 25 24 23 22   1 2 3 4 5

This book is also available as an eBook.

ABC-CLIO
An Imprint of ABC-CLIO, LLC

ABC-CLIO, LLC
147 Castilian Drive
Santa Barbara, California 93117
www.abc-clio.com

This book is printed on acid-free paper ∞

Manufactured in the United States of America

Contents

How to Use This Book

Vaccination: Examining the Facts is part of ABC-CLIO's "Contemporary Debates" reference series. Each title in this series, which is intended for use by high school and undergraduate students as well as members of the general public, examines the veracity of controversial claims or beliefs surrounding a major political/cultural issue in the United States. The purpose of this series is to give readers a clear, unbiased understanding of current issues by informing them about falsehoods, half-truths, and misconceptions—and confirming the factual validity of other assertions—that have gained traction in the United States' political and cultural discourse. Ultimately, this series has been crafted to give readers the tools for a fuller understanding of controversial issues, policies, and laws that occupy center stage in U.S. life and politics.

Each volume in this series identifies 30 to 40 questions swirling about the larger topic under discussion. These questions are examined in individualized entries, which are in turn arranged in broad subject chapters that cover certain aspects of the issue being examined, for example, history of concern about the issue, potential economic or social impact, or findings of the latest scholarly research.

Each chapter features 4 to 10 individual entries. Each entry begins by stating an important and/or well-known **Question** about the issue being studied—for example, "Do vaccines prevent disease?" and "Do we know where COVID-19 came from?" and "Is vaccine misinformation dangerous?"

The entry then provides a concise, objective one- or two-paragraph **Answer** to the featured question, followed by a more comprehensive, detailed explanation of **The Facts**. This latter portion of each entry uses quantifiable, evidence-based information from respected sources to fully address each question and provide readers with the information they need to be informed citizens. Importantly, entries will also acknowledge instances in which conflicting or incomplete data exists or legal judgments are contradictory. Finally, each entry concludes with a **Further Reading** section, providing users with information on other important or influential resources.

The ultimate purpose of every book in the "Contemporary Debates" series is to reject "false equivalence," in which demonstrably false beliefs or statements are given the same exposure and credence as the facts; to puncture myths that diminish our understanding of important policies and positions; to provide needed context for misleading statements and claims; and to confirm the factual accuracy of other assertions. In other words, volumes in this series are being crafted to clear the air surrounding some of the most contentious and misunderstood issues or our time—not just add another layer of obfuscation and uncertainty to the debate.

Introduction

In a book filled with questions, one question stands out: What is the best way to protect individuals, families, communities, nations, and entire populations from infectious diseases? The answer is vaccines. It is a science-based, time-tested answer, founded on three centuries of vaccination programs that have saved the lives and ensured the futures of millions of men, women, and children. Vaccination is also a routine part of livestock care that has been used on millions of animals that form part of the human ecosystem, thus ensuring food supply and agricultural production for people who rely on them.

Vaccines administered from 2000 through 2019 are estimated to have averted 50 million deaths. Vaccines are estimated to be on track to prevent another 47 million deaths by 2030 (Toor, 2021). This count does not include the COVID-19 vaccine, which was estimated by one study to have saved 279,000 lives and prevented 1.25 million hospitalizations in its first six months of administration in the United States alone (Gray, 2021).

With a track record so successful, we might think that vaccination programs, like clean water or clean air, would be something everyone can agree on. But health care decisions are often complex, and although people who are hesitant or opposed to vaccines have always been in the minority, they have always been part of the conversation. Health care experts who recognize that fact assert that the best way to move forward in search of common ground and understanding is to keep the conversation fact-based, so that it is not overwhelmed by political or social agendas.

Vaccination: Examining the Facts is my contribution to the discussion. I first began in work on it in the fall of 2019, but the eruption of the COVID-19 pandemic into my life, and that of the community, country, and world around me, completely changed my conception of the book I wanted to write. In January and February 2020, we began hearing about the new infectious disease spreading so rapidly across the world. I can no longer recall the date when we recognized that the question was no longer if, but when, it would reach my community in the northeastern United States. By mid-March 2020, we were in lockdown. I found myself in the midst of events I had studied as a historian of medicine, our experiences mirroring those of the characters in Daniel Defoe's *Journal of the Plague Year* and the 2011 movie *Contagion*. We followed COVID-19 case trackers as Defoe's narrator followed the London Bills of Mortality; we hoped and prayed for a vaccine, as did the protagonists in *Contagion*.

The issues that I had taught in my college courses for many years were the subject of frequent, sometimes daily interrogation in news and social media as well as professional and scholarly journals. What were vaccines? How effective were they, and how could we be sure they were safe? If they were so wonderful, why didn't we have them for all diseases? Why was it so much easier for rich people to get health care than poor people? What could be done to close the gap between vaccine-have and vaccine-have-not communities, both in the United States and around the globe? If people knew—as they had for decades—that vaccine-preventable diseases were only a plane ride away, then why hadn't more been done to protect vulnerable populations from danger?

The COVID-19 pandemic brought its own pressing questions. Could vaccines be developed quickly enough to stem the pandemic, and if so, would they be safe? How could they be distributed worldwide? Would crime disrupt supply chains? Would vaccine hesitancy disrupt a vaccine rollout? Was it possible to stem the tide of misinformation that threatened public health measures in the United States and across the world? Would any of the lessons learned from the impact of COVID-19 be remembered during other, future public health crises?

This book, then, was very much written through the lens of COVID-19. That doesn't mean I have neglected the insights gleaned from other vaccine-preventable diseases. As a historian, I believe that lessons from the past are essential in allowing us to chart a path toward the future. But I believe that a key lesson of the COVID-19 pandemic is that we cannot allow ourselves to be complacent. We must accept the science-based fact that vaccine-preventable diseases, both those we already know and those we will encounter in the future, will always be extremely dangerous to our lives and well-being if we cannot or will not make use of the vaccines that prevent them.

This book is divided into five sections. The first, *How do vaccines work*, deals with the science of vaccines and the safety and efficacy of vaccination programs. The second is *Vaccines to the rescue: The COVID-19 pandemic and vaccine development*. It focuses on the many different stakeholders worked together and separately to manufacture and distribute COVID-19 vaccines, and the many challenges they faced. The third is *Key issues in global vaccination*, which looks at the progress made—and remaining roadblocks to progress—in expanding global access to vaccines that wealthy nations take for granted. The fourth is *Vaccination controversies*. While providing insight into historical controversies, this section focuses more on areas of contention that emerged during the pandemic, including the role of social media in spreading disinformation and legal questions concerning vaccine mandates. The fifth section, *Vaccines for a healthier future*, looks at the lessons learned from the past half-century, and particularly the past three years, of vaccination research, development, and distribution. Few experts think COVID-19 will be our last infectious disease outbreak. But if we learn from the COVID-19 pandemic, perhaps we will be able to keep it our last vaccine-preventable global health care crisis.

A fact-based history of vaccines contains many cautionary tales, but it also contains much hope and inspiration. This book is dedicated to the many health care heroes whose hard work, good sense, and dedication kept us all going during the COVID-19 pandemic. I hope it may serve as a reference, and perhaps an inspiration, for the next generation of heroes.

FURTHER READING

Gray, Sidney. 2021. "YSPH Study Finds COVID-19 Vaccine Rollout Has Saved 279,000 Lives." *Yale Daily News*. https://yaledailynews.com /blog/2021/09/02/ysph-study-finds-covid-19-vaccine-rollout-has -saved-279000-lives/.

Toor, Japrit, et al. 2021. "Lives Saved with Vaccination for 10 Pathogens across 112 Countries in a Pre-COVID-19 World." *eLifeSciences*. https:// elifesciences.org/articles/67635.

1

❖

How Do Vaccines Work?

INTRODUCTION

This section explores the most basic questions about vaccines: how they work, how they strengthen the body's immune system, and how they have been used to eradicate and eliminate disease in human populations and in those of the animals they depend upon. Vaccination policies and regulations are embedded in modern health care practices in the United States and around the globe. It's too much to say that they act as a force field, so that all potentially infectious diseases bounce off when they get close to human targets. However, it is entirely accurate to say that vaccines, and the policies and programs that regulate and distribute them, act as an interlocking set of security systems to deflect known disease threats against humans and animals. In humans alone, vaccines are estimated to prevent between four and five million deaths each year. They are estimated to avert over $800 billion in health care costs throughout the world.

In some ways, modern vaccine technologies are like modern transportation technologies, such as automobiles, trains, and planes. One similarity is that people seldom think much about them until they need them. Few people pay much attention to the details of vaccines unless they need them for school, work, or their children, in the same way that few people pay attention to how their cars work, or to the mechanics of trains or airplanes.

Yet another similarity is that there is continuous research and development in vaccine manufacturing, testing, regulation, and distribution, just as there is in transportation networks. The vaccines currently available are far more effective and sophisticated than the earliest smallpox inoculations of the 18th century, just as a Boeing 787 Dreamliner is far beyond the Wright Brothers airplane flown in 1903, and a Tesla far beyond an 18th-century horse-drawn cart. Modern vaccines have been built on centuries of scientific research and evaluation, making use of advances in medicine, new technologies, and the most recent data.

Another similarity is that people take for granted that vaccines, like the cars, trains, and planes, will be there when they need them. That means they take for granted the science and public policy behind vaccine development, regulation, manufacture, and distribution, just as they take for granted that there will be roads available to them when they drive their cars, and train stations and airports waiting for them when they need to take a train or plane. Most people only notice the infrastructure necessary when there's a problem: vaccines that are unavailable or inaccessible, potholes on highways, delays in train or airplane travel. And the best solution, for vaccines as well as for transportation, is to try to avoid having the problems arise. That involves advance planning by scientific experts, including physicians, research scientists, engineers, and systems analysts.

A final similarity between vaccine programs and transportation networks is the importance of consumer protection and advocacy necessary for both. For vaccination programs to be acceptable to the modern world, every single vaccine must be demonstrated to work against its targeted disease. It must be rigorously tested and certified according to the highest possible standards for safety. And it must be accessible, so that it is available to everyone who needs it without delay. These are the same consumer standards we apply to transportation networks such as highways, rail lines, and air routes, and also to the cars, trains, and planes that run on them.

In vaccine science, as in so much else, the best consumer is an educated consumer. This first chapter will help readers chart their path toward becoming educated, knowledgeable consumers of vaccines and vaccination policies. Many other trustworthy sources can be found online. The Centers for Disease Control and Prevention (CDC) provides an excellent overview for U.S. immunization practices, in addition to guidance for federal, state, and local public health policy (https://www.cdc.gov/vaccines/index.html). The World Health Organization (WHO), which considers vaccination a human right, provides information and guidance on global policy and practices (https://www.who.int/health-topics/vaccines-and-immunization). The United Nations Children's Fund (UNICEF) is another authoritative source: UNICEF vaccinates 45 percent of the world's children under five years old, more than any other single organization (https://www.unicef.org/immunization).

The information provided in this section and in external trustworthy sources is the basis for the most up-to-date vaccine practices and policies in the modern world. It will help readers understand key issues discussed in the remaining sections of this book. It provides context for the many health care debates that received national and international attention during the COVID-19 pandemic and sheds light on issues crucial to public health policy decision-making, both now and for decades to come.

Q1. DO VACCINES PREVENT DISEASE?

Answer: Yes. A vaccine is a biological substance that trains the immune system to detect and protect against microorganisms that cause disease. These microorganisms come in two broad classes, bacteria and viruses, and a specific vaccine will guard against a specific bacterium or virus. For example, anthrax vaccines protect people and livestock against the disease of anthrax, caused by a type of bacteria called *Bacillus anthracis*. The COVID-19 vaccine protects people against the disease caused by a specific virus, severe acute respiratory syndrome coronavirus 2 (SARS-CoV-2). The process of administering vaccines is known as vaccination or immunization. Though the best-known immunizations are intended for children, many adults benefit from immunizations as well.

Vaccines serve two key purposes: they protect individual people from catching a dangerous disease, and they stop the spread of that disease within the general population.

The Facts: The battle to protect individuals and groups from external infectious agents, often called pathogens or germs, has sometimes been compared to a version of a Space Invaders videogame. Pathogens are always out there in the world, but to actually get to individual human bodies, they have to pass through a number of barriers.

The first is the protective barrier provided by communities in the modern world. These include water and sewage treatments that destroy disease-causing pathogens, processes like pasteurization that do the same for dairy products, and standards for the safety and quality of food sold in stores. It also includes certain kinds of social behaviors, like washing hands after using the toilet or wearing gloves and masks to protect against the spread of disease. This community public health infrastructure has evolved in response to epidemic diseases that attacked human populations in the past. Cholera, for example, spreads through water, so water treatment programs that kill cholera help keep people from ever encountering the bacillus that causes it. If this were a game, you could think of these barriers as a kind of long-range missile that can be deployed to attack and destroy certain kinds of infectious pathogens before they even reach people.

The second protection is the protective barrier of the human skin, mucous membranes, and the beneficial microorganisms that block a range of external agents, including dust or chemicals as well as germs. If this were a game, this would be a screen with very small openings, perfectly shaped to fit the human body and protect it from dangerous substances.

The third barrier is the activity of white blood cells called phagocytes. When there is a break in the skin, such as a cut or bruise, and pathogens— usually bacteria—enter the body, the body responds with a process called inflammation, with symptoms including redness and swelling around the cut or bruise. The inflammation triggers the deployment of phagocytes, which attack foreign substances that enter the body. Phagocytes, however, can't be tailored to defend against specific pathogens. If this were a game, these would be the standard weapons used to defend the planet: they can be deployed against any microorganisms, but they can't adapt to new conditions. If a pathogen can evolve to evade the phagocytes, or to attack them directly, then they are no longer an effective defense.

The fourth protective barrier is the defense mechanism known as adaptive immunity. This is the function of the immune system, one of the most complex systems of the human body, with more than 1,600 genes involved in its functions. Every person's immune system is immature at birth, and newborns rely at first on the immune response transferred at birth from their mothers. From birth until old age, the human immune system is constantly learning to recognize and develop defenses against diseases. Some of these threats are very rare, such as Histoplasmosis, an infection spread by pigeon droppings. Some are very familiar, such as the common cold. Some are infectious, like measles. In each of these cases, the immune system learns to recognize that specific microorganism that causes the disease, develops mechanisms to destroy it, and then remembers those mechanisms when the microorganism attacks again. In a game, these would be the most intelligent of the defensive weapons marshalled against invaders. Not only can they be trained to recognize and protect against specific pathogens, but they can also be trained to remember the pathogens the next time they invade, and redeploy in the body's defense.

The problem with these "adaptive immunity" defenses, as they are sometimes called, is that some disease pathogens can overwhelm the defenses that people were born with. That means that people who contract those diseases are at a high risk of getting sick and even dying. The people and communities they live with are also at a high risk of catching the disease from them and, in turn, spreading it to others.

Scientists who study the spread of disease, known as epidemiologists, call the number of patients who contract the disease in a given population the morbidity rate or the rate of infection of that disease. They may also refer to the number of patients who test positive, meaning that patients have been tested for the disease and found to be carrying it. This information may be calculated as "cases per 1,000" or "cases per million." For COVID-19, there were 136,999 cases per million in the United States (which has a total population of about 328 million) from January 2020 through October 2021. The total number of people who caught COVID-19 during that time period was 45.6 million. These are measures of morbidity based on the U.S. population as a whole; they varied widely by region and by demographic factors such as race and age.

Epidemiologists call the rate at which patients die from a specific disease the mortality or fatality rate. The population fatality rate is the number of patients who die throughout the total population being studied. It includes both people who have contracted the disease and those who have not. The case fatality rate is the number of patients who die after contracting the disease. Between January and August 2020, the U.S. population fatality rate for COVID-19 was 578 per million, or 189,000 total. The case fatality rate was 3 percent, meaning that 3 percent of patients who caught the disease later died from it.

Three percent may not seem like a lot, but it can quickly add up. Imagine, for example, a class or meeting room that holds 33 people—and now imagine millions of classrooms that size across the United States. A 3 percent case fatality rate means that one person in each room would die. In rooms that were filled with older people—adults over age 60—or people with preexisting health conditions, like diabetes, even more patients would die. Thanks to adaptive immunity, it is likely that people who recovered would not get it again. But it would still keep spreading to new populations, including the millions of babies born between each new outbreak.

That was exactly the situation in which people lived before the 20th century, a time when dangerous diseases like smallpox, with a 30 percent case fatality rate, or diphtheria, with a 5–10 percent case fatality rate, stalked the world. Less developed transportation networks limited the severity and number of epidemics—severe outbreaks—or pandemics—worldwide outbreaks. In the 21st century, though, any new disease that develops anywhere in the world is a plane ride away from spreading across the rest of the globe.

For thousands of years, individual people and communities have harnessed human ingenuity to combat these deadly diseases. In the past 300 years, especially, we have developed ways to study microorganisms on their own terms, so we can create vaccines to prevent them from causing and spreading disease.

A specific vaccine gives the body's immune system a small taste of what it would be like to get a specific disease, so human adaptive immunity can store that memory and deploy it when the disease comes along in full force. Vaccines build on, strengthen, and extend the reach of the adaptive immunity we are born with. In our Space Invaders game, vaccines are our ultimate defense: they are specific weapons that recognize and combat a specific pathogen whenever it appears.

In the United States, immunizations are currently used to prevent 27 diseases, including COVID-19. Once we have been vaccinated for them, we carry that immunity around with us for long periods of time—for some diseases, our entire lifespan. This immunity works like a two-pronged force field: it protects individuals from getting the disease, and it ensures that we won't spread it to anyone else. Scientists estimate, for example, that more than 279,000 lives were saved by the COVID-19 vaccine between December 2020 and October 2021.

Certain types of vaccine-preventable diseases are often known as childhood diseases, including smallpox, mumps, measles, and diphtheria. This is not because only children can get them, but because they are so infectious that they spread rapidly to any vulnerable population. Before there were vaccines to prevent them, these diseases were endemic—that is, always present in the population—in many parts of the world. Most people got them when they were very young, and they either recovered or died. If they recovered, they developed an immunity to the disease and so were no longer vulnerable as adults.

If an infectious disease spreads to a new, vulnerable community full of members who had never been exposed to it, then people of any age can catch it. When smallpox, measles, and influenza spread from Europeans to Native Americans in the 17th and 18th centuries, the mortality rate for Native Americans was extraordinarily high among all ages. For tribes in some regions, the mortality rate was estimated at 90 percent of the population. On the Yamal peninsula in Siberia, anthrax had not been seen since the last outbreak in 1941, and families assumed it had been eradicated—that is, it was no longer present in the population. But conditions of melting ice, caused by global warming, led to the reawakening of anthrax spores buried in an infected reindeer during that 1941 outbreak. In 2016, several thousand reindeer were infected by a new outbreak, as were dozens of people from reindeer-herding families. One 12-year-old boy died, and the infected herds had to be destroyed—tragic family and economic outcomes for the district.

Vaccines should be distinguished from other ways of dealing with disease, such as treatments and cures. A treatment is anything that is given to a patient to help reduce the symptoms and effects of a disease. This might include bed rest to keep the patient comfortable and protect other people from catching the disease. Another common treatment is medication such as painkillers, designed to relieve fever and pain, or medicines to help the body's own immune system fight the disease. It might also include more intensive equipment, like intravenous (IV) therapy to introduce fluids or medications directly into the vein, or ventilators to help patients get sufficient oxygen. Treatment can also refer to medications that directly target microorganisms, like antibiotics, or that have other biological impacts, such as insulin medication for controlling diabetes. The term "cures," as the name implies, refers to treatments that are known to effect a cure.

Vaccines help prevent diseases by strengthening and extending the body's immune system. The pathogen is destroyed before it can attack vulnerable cells and replicate. Once the pathogen has already made it past the immune system, so that the patient already has the disease, vaccines are no longer effective. For that reason, vaccines should be given before an individual is exposed to the disease. The pathogens for some diseases, like rabies, are very slow to reach the part of the body they have evolved to attack, so the rabies vaccine can still be effective even if given after the patient has been infected by a bite from an animal with rabies. But most other infectious diseases invade the body and spread so quickly that by the time patients show symptoms, the vaccine will no longer be effective. As the saying goes, an ounce of prevention is worth a pound of cure.

FURTHER READING

Centers for Disease Control and Prevention. n.d. "Vaccines by Disease." Accessed January 25, 2021. https://www.cdc.gov/vaccines/vpd/vaccines -list.html.

Centers for Disease Control and Prevention. n.d. "Vaccinations by Age." Accessed January 25, 2021. https://www.cdc.gov/vaccines/vpd/vaccines -age.html.

Diamond, Jared. 1999. *Guns Germs and Steel: The Fates of Human Societies*. New York: W. W. Norton and Company.

Fox-Skelly, Jasmin. 2017. "There Are Diseases Hidden in Ice, and They Are Waking Up." BBC, May 4, 2017. http://www.bbc.co.uk/earth

/story/20170504-there-are-diseases-hidden-in-ice-and-they-are
-waking-up.

Simon, A. Katharina, Georg A. Hollander, and Andrew McMichael. 2015.
"Evolution of the Immune System in Humans from Infancy to Old Age."
Proceedings of the Biological Society, 282, 1821 (2015): 20143085. https://
www.ncbi.nlm.nih.gov/pmc/articles/PMC4707740/.

Q2. DO VACCINES HELP STRENGTHEN THE BODY'S NATURAL DEFENSES?

Answer: Yes. Vaccines work directly with the components of the body's own immune system. using the same types of biochemical mechanisms. They induce the immune system to manufacture a specific set of molecules, known as antibodies, to combat the pathogens that cause disease. It's helpful to think of each type of antibody as a highly specialized, made-to-order tool that attaches itself to the pathogen, either weakening it or destroying it. The immune system's own biochemical processes will manufacture the same tools if it comes into contact with the disease—but that can be very risky if the disease itself is dangerous. Vaccines work with the body to increase the range of the immune system's protective tool kit, but without the risk of death or other serious outcomes.

Humans generate about 10 billion different antibodies, and the more antibodies the immune system can produce, the better defense it can provide. Vaccines thus build up and strengthen the body's natural defenses against disease in much the same way that weight training and other physical exercise strengthen the body's natural muscular response, speed, and endurance.

The Facts: In order to understand how vaccines work, we can start by looking at the immune system, which is the body's natural defense against disease and injury. When people or animals get sick, the disease affects their entire body. However, the mechanism by which they get sick is best understood at the cellular level. The microorganism, or specialized parts of it, attack the cells of its host—that is, the infected person or animal. Once a pathogen cell infects a body cell, it will spread from cell to cell, infecting one after another until it is stopped. It is the job of the immune system to deploy its own specialized sets of protective cells to repel the invaders.

The human immune system is very highly developed and effective. Any detection of foreign cells—external invading cells that are not part of the body—triggers a protective response from white blood cells (leukocytes).

The precise molecules, or molecular structures, on the foreign cells that trigger the response are known as antigens. Antigens may be made of complex protein molecules, or they may be made of lipids (fat molecules) or polysaccharides (sugar molecules). In addition to announcing the presence of the pathogen, they may also be part of the biochemical mechanism that helps the disease attack the body.

The "spike" so often depicted in images of the cell of SARS-CoV-2 (the virus that causes COVID-19) is a good example of an antigen. It both signals the immune system that COVID-19 is present, and it provides the mechanism by which the disease attaches itself to cells in the human body. The so-called spike doesn't literally have a sharp point like a metal spike. Instead, it is built out of proteins with a particular molecular shape. Those proteins attach themselves to a specific type of receptor proteins, known as ACE2, with a molecular shape that makes it vulnerable to the protein spike. ACE2 receptors are found on the surface of many types of body cells but are particularly common in the respiratory tract. Once the antigens on the surface of COVID-19 cells have attached themselves to the ACE2 receptors of human cells, they have a pathway to enter and infect the cell itself. That is, of course, dangerous to the human whose cells are being attacked.

Fortunately, the immune system has evolved to protect against exactly that kind of attack. Once the immune system detects an antigen, it begins its own series of biochemical processes to mount a defense. Each type of white blood cell has its own task. Antigen-presenting cells (APCs) ingest the invading antigen and process it so that a piece of the antigen is displayed on the APC's surface. The APC cells then travel to sites in the body where white blood cells are manufactured, such as the lymph nodes. When they come into contact with another type of white blood cell called T cells, some of the T cells become activated into helper T cells. These T helper cells notify nearby cells of the presence of the invading antigen by secreting cytokines, a type of chemical messenger.

The presence of cytokines activates another type of white blood cell, B cells. Once activated, B cells quickly produce two subtypes: memory B cells and plasma B cells. A memory B cell "remembers" the specific type of antigen that triggered it. That is, if the same antigen appears again, it will provoke the same set of defense mechanisms. Plasma B cells generate antibodies to attack and either weaken or destroy the invading antigen. Both memory B cells and plasma B cells are produced in response to a specific antigen and will only be effective against that antigen. That is why an antibody produced in response to the flu, for example, will not work against COVID-19. It's helpful to think of B cells, and the resulting antibodies, as extremely specialized, microscopic tools to do an extremely specialized task in protecting the body.

The antibodies produced by the plasma B cells are another type of protein, and they are usually depicted with a distinctive "Y" shape. The actual shape, on the molecular level, is adapted to fit the molecules on the antigen that triggered them. Huge numbers of antibodies are released per second, and they bind themselves tightly to the antigen in what is usually described as a "lock and key" mechanism. This action can make it impossible for the antigen to enter a healthy cell, and it can also mark the antigen as an invading cell, so that it can be easily detected and destroyed.

The cytokines generated by helper T cells also trigger the production of two more specialized type of T cell, killer (or cytotoxic) T cells and memory T cells. Killer T cells, as the name implies, directly attack the invading pathogen cells and any cells the pathogen has infected. They can travel throughout the body and attack a wide range of toxic invasive cells. Memory T cells serve a similar purpose as the memory B cells: they allow the immune system to "remember" and keep track of a specific invading antigen, so that they can respond quickly if they encounter it again.

Though all these types of cells can seem confusing, the key point is that they work as a highly effective defense team, with a first line of response designed to quickly destroy the invaders, followed by long-term strategy to repel them if they ever turn up again. When we get sick, our first experience of it may include fever, coughing, diarrhea, and vomiting. These are all mechanisms by which our bodies try to immediately kill an invading pathogen— no matter what the pathogen is. While that's going on, the more specialized parts of our immune system kick into high gear. Our ordinary, nonspecific (often called naive) T and B cells rapidly proliferate into specialized plasma B cells to produce millions of targeted antibodies (and killer T cells) to attack the specific pathogen. That same process produces millions of memory B and memory T cells, ensuring that if the same disease tries to invade our cells again, the immune system will recognize it even more rapidly and start generating antibodies and killer T cells before the pathogen can have any impact. As the millions of antibodies in our bodies attest, in most cases the immune system can repel the invading pathogens, protecting us before we even know we have come into contact with the disease.

Although the immune system is highly effective, it's not perfect. A particularly dangerous pathogen can overwhelm the body's defenses, leading to serious symptoms and death. The good news is that even dangerous pathogens can exist in many strains, some of which are less virulent—that is, they are less dangerous to the body—than others. It turns out that the immune system will produce the same antibodies for a weak strain as for a strong one, and the memory B and T cells it produces can be just as effective in guarding against future disease.

The principle that having a mild version of a disease can protect people against a more dangerous version of it has been known for thousands of years. It is the basis for the medical knowledge, already well documented in the ancient world, that children who recover from a mild version of potentially deadly infectious diseases like smallpox or diphtheria can't get it again, even if exposed to very virulent strains of it.

The fact that recovering from a mild version of a large number of serious infectious diseases conveys immunity to that disease was the basis for the earliest inoculation practices, documented in China and the Mediterranean by the 1500s and available in western Europe and the Americas by the 1700s. In this early form of inoculation, medical practitioners artificially produced a mild case of smallpox in children and adults, in order to protect them against deadlier strains. On the cellular level, this triggered the rapid-response system of white blood cells to first, destroy the invading smallpox cells, and second, create memory B and T cells to ward off future invasions.

Modern vaccines have become much more sophisticated, but they still rely on the body's own natural defenses. They rely on the patient being injected with—or, in some cases, swallowing—an antigen that has been found, through rigorous research, to trigger the immune response. Historically, vaccines have been either a weakened or inactivated version of the original pathogen.

For COVID-19, two of the vaccines use a different approach based on up-to-date research on genomes, which is the genetic material found in a cell. The vaccines inject messenger RNA (mRNA) into the body, where it connects to cells and provides instructions on manufacturing the distinctive protein spike. The instructions only produce the spike, not the invading pathogen. That is, the vaccine doesn't inject or generate the actual SARS-CoV-2 virus cells, which means that patients can't get COVID-19 from the vaccine. Once it has conveyed its instructions, the mRNA is destroyed as part of the cell's natural metabolic process. Some of the spike proteins are conveyed to the cell's surface, as part of that same process. When the cell dies, additional protein spikes or parts of spikes are released and travel to the lymph nodes.

At that point the rest of the immune system kicks in. The vaccine-induced protein spikes are antigens, so antigen-presenting cells detect them. They activate T and B cells. The former produce helper T cells, and then killer T and memory T cells. The latter produce B plasma—which in turn produce antibodies—and B memory cells. By the end of the process, the antigen trigger—the protein spikes—have all been destroyed, and the immune system has a molecular "memory" of their biochemical shape. Should any subsequent SARS-CoV-2 virus cells attempt to invade, the immune system will immediately produce antibodies to defend against them.

Vaccines ensure that the body is primed and ready when exposed to actual diseases. This is especially important when a disease is infectious and potentially deadly. When people who are protected by vaccines come in contact with the pathogen, they may well breathe in, or swallow, the invading cells. However, the antigens on those cells will quickly trigger the APCs. The APCs will immediately activate memory T cells, which instantly recognize the antigen. The memory T cells go straight to activating the memory B cells for that antigen, and those memory B cells differentiate into plasma B cells. The plasma B cells ramp up the secretion of antibodies, providing even more of them, even more quickly, than in the original response.

A similar speeded-up process extends to T cells: the memory helper T cells move straight to the production of killer T cells in order to destroy the invading pathogen and any infected cells. The vaccine thus works with the body's immune system to protect the individual from the disease. As the vaccine speeds up the immune response, the rapid destruction of the pathogen cells by antibodies and killer T cells helps prevent the individual from infecting anyone else.

FURTHER READING

Allen, Arthur. *Vaccine. The Controversial Story of Medicine's Greatest Lifesaver.* 2007. New York: W. W. Norton & Company.

Corum, Jonathan, and Carl Zimmer. 2021a. "How Moderna's Vaccine Works." *New York Times*, January 11, 2021, https://www.nytimes.com/interactive/2020/health/moderna-covid-19-vaccine.html.

Corum, Jonathan, and Carl Zimmer. 2021b. "How the Pfizer-BioNTech Vaccine Works." *New York Times*, January 11, 2021, https://www.nytimes.com/interactive/2020/health/pfizer-biontech-covid-19-vaccine.html.

History of Vaccines. n.d. "How Vaccines Work." Accessed January 25, 2021. https://www.historyofvaccines.org/content/how-vaccines-work.

MacDonald, Anna. 2017. "Antigen vs Antibody—What Are the Differences?" *Technology Networks.* https://www.technologynetworks.com/immunology/articles/antigen-vs-antibody-what-are-the-differences-293550.

Zimmer, Carl. 2020. "The Coronavirus Unveiled." *New York Times*. https://www.nytimes.com/interactive/2020/health/coronavirus-unveiled.html.

Q3. DO VACCINES CAUSE SIDE EFFECTS?

Answer: Yes. A side effect is any effect other than the intended medical purpose, and side effects are common to many types of medical prevention and treatment. Most people understand the term "side effects" to have negative connotations, but some forms of medical prevention and cure can have positive side effects. For example, the smallpox vaccine was found to protect at least some patients against other kinds of infections as well. For all modern vaccines, side effects are carefully monitored as part of the vaccine approval process. They usually affect fewer than 10 percent of the patients who receive the vaccine.

Vaccines given as injections may produce two types of side effects: local and systemic. Local side effects are those that affect the injection site but appear nowhere else on the patient. They may include pain, redness, and swelling around the point of the injection. Systemic side effects are those that affect the whole body and may include fever, headache, and chills. Both types of side effects *resolve*, or go away, within one to three days. Though often unpleasant when they appear, they should be seen as important signs that the vaccine is working as intended.

Serious vaccine side effects are rare compared to food allergies. Approximately 11 percent of the adult population of the United States reports some form of food allergy, and 38 percent of those have ended up in hospital emergency rooms due to those allergies. Severe allergic and other reactions to vaccination are approximately 1 in 1,000,000, or .0001 percent.

The Facts: Patients and their health care professionals would much prefer that vaccines came with no side effects, as it would make it much more pleasant to get them. As Dr. Paul Offit, director of the Vaccine Education Center at the Children's Hospital of Philadelphia, put it, "I wish the immune system had a better PR team" (Lewis, 2020). What he means is that it would be much easier on everyone if the vaccines that enhance the effectiveness of the immune system also made patients feel good right away. After all, our expectation of modern medication is that drugs or other treatments should make us feel better, not worse. If we take a painkiller, we expect it to relieve pain. If we suffer from high cholesterol or diabetes, we expect the medication prescribed for those health issues to allow us to live a healthier, more active lifestyle.

The activity of the immune system in response to vaccination is not directed against the patient but rather against the perceived intruder pathogen. The local redness, pain, and swelling that many people experience after receiving a shot is the healthy response of the body to the invading antigen as well as the puncture wound caused by the injection. The symptoms are part of the natural healing process, which is why they go away so quickly. Local pain and swelling, as well as fever, chills, and headaches, are all part of the immune system's efforts to destroy invading pathogens by increasing the body temperature. They are not an indication that anything has gone wrong or that the patient has contracted the disease. Instead, they are the business-as-usual immune response, and they go away much more quickly than the actual disease.

Concern about side effects is, in its way, a side effect of improvements in modern medicine. During the 19th century, many patients preferred to take medicine that was bad-tasting, strong-smelling, and produced noticeable effects in the body, like vomiting. They believed that the more dangerous the disease, the stronger the medicine had to be in order to act against it. When simple pills without taste, smell, or impact on the digestive system were introduced in the early 20th century, older patients found it difficult to believe that they worked. Nowadays, medication that causes nausea as a side effect is considered to be acceptable only for very serious illnesses, such as chemotherapy for cancer treatment. It is certainly not considered to be a desirable feature, and therapies are available to reduce the nausea associated with modern cancer treatments.

Side effects also loom larger in popular medical ideas because few people have had firsthand experience of patients with serious vaccine-preventable diseases. Diphtheria, for example, used to be a serious infectious disease that mostly struck young children. The symptoms included high fever; a thick, whitish covering of the back of the throat that made it hard for sufferers to breathe or swallow; sore throat; nausea; and vomiting. The mortality rate in a severe diphtheria epidemic could get up to one patient in seven (about 14%). In contrast, the side effects of the diphtheria vaccine are the usual local effects of redness, pain, and swelling at the site of the injection and a mild fever, which goes away within a day or two. These mild side effects appear in only one out of 10 patients receiving the diphtheria vaccine. Patients who had experienced diphtheria outbreaks, or who knew about them from older relatives, showed little concern about vaccination side effects. They recognized that even if they were sore or even feverish after the injection, they were still avoiding the risk of much more severe health risks if they caught the disease.

The same is true for many other diseases. Seven out of ten adult patients with hepatitis A develop extremely unpleasant symptoms, including jaundice, liver pain, fever, nausea, and vomiting. They lose their appetite and have a hard time keeping food down when they do eat. If they get the vaccine, on the other hand, they may only feel some redness, pain, and swelling at the vaccination site.

Pertussis, which leads to the condition known as whooping cough, is distressing at any age, but it is especially dangerous for babies under the age of six months. About one out of 125 babies (.8%) who contract pertussis end up dying from pneumonia or brain damage. The side effects of the vaccine consist of the usual pain, redness, and swelling at the vaccination site and mild fever; these temporary side effects appear in approximately one out of 10 vaccinated babies (10%).

The side effects associated with the COVID-19 vaccines were very carefully studied. They were found to be the usual ones associated with the immune response: pain, redness, and swelling at the vaccination site, as well as fever, headache, and chills. Patients who reported side effects found they were more severe after the second shot of the Pfizer and Moderna vaccines than after the first. Older patients over the age of 65 were less likely to report side effects than those 64 years old and younger.

For the Moderna vaccine, between 80 and 90 percent of patients reported some local reaction, most frequently pain and redness. The pain was reported in some cases as severe enough to prevent activity or for the patient to take over-the-counter pain medication. It was not so severe as to warrant a trip to the doctor or emergency room. Systemic reactions were less common, but those who experienced them were more likely to do so after the second dose. Approximately 50 percent of people receiving the Moderna vaccine reported some sort of systemic side effect, with approximately 30 percent experiencing fatigue and headache severe enough to require pain medication. In the younger group, 18 percent reported fever, and in the older group, 10 percent reported it. The side effects disappeared after one to two days.

The most serious side effect for any vaccine is an allergic reaction, because it can lead to anaphylaxis, a severe overreaction on the part of the immune system, which can lead to shock and, if left untreated, death. It is the same type of reaction that affects patients with allergies to peanuts or bee stings. It can be treated through the immediate injection of epinephrine, but treatment must be administered right away.

Because anaphylaxis is a well-known, though rare, response to vaccination, vaccine researchers made sure to allow for it during vaccine administration. Patients are prescreened to see if they have a history of allergic reactions. Because allergic reactions usually show up very rapidly, provisions are made for patients to stay at the vaccination site for at least 15 minutes after receiving the injection. The estimated rates of anaphylaxis after COVID-19 vaccination are 2.8 to 5.0 per million doses. These cases were caught before they became life-threatening, and all were treated successfully.

Clinical trials and firsthand accounts show how important it is for patients to know about side effects in advance, so they are not surprised or alarmed when they appear. Dr. Kristin Choi, a registered nurse, described her own experience as a volunteer for the Pfizer COVID-19 vaccine clinical trials. The trials were double-blind studies, in which neither participants nor health care workers knew who would get the actual vaccine and who would get a "placebo," a harmless substance without any antigens. Choi therefore did not know whether she was given the vaccine or the placebo. After the first shot, she only experienced some soreness in her arm, which she might have expected in either case. It was only after the second shot that she experienced side effects—and, as she described, they were both uncomfortable and frightening. "My arm quickly became painful at the injection site," she recalled, "much more than the first time. By the end of the day, I felt light-headed, chilled, nauseous, and had a splitting headache. I went to bed early and fell asleep immediately. . . . When I woke up again at 5:30 a.m., I felt hot. Burning. I took my temperature and looked at the reading: 104.9°F. This was the highest fever I can ever remember having, and it scared me." Choi took over-the-counter pain medication, and by the next day, her symptoms had disappeared, except for "a sore, swollen bump on the injection site." That also disappeared over the next 24 hours.

Although she was an experienced nurse researcher herself, Choi noted that "on a personal level I did not get the message that I should anticipate" side effects. She was reassured to learn that other participants of the trials had experienced side effects, and as she later found out, most people's side effects had been much milder than her own. She recommended that all health professionals be honest with their patients about the possibility of side effects (Choi, 2020). Although telling patients what to expect does not keep the side effects from happening, it does let them know that though uncomfortable, they are a by-product of the natural functioning of the immune system. These conversations increase patient confidence that their immune systems, the vaccine, and health care professionals are all doing their jobs to protect their health.

FURTHER READING

Centers for Disease Control and Prevention. 2021. "Allergic Reactions Including Anaphylaxis after Receipt of the First Dose of Pfizer-BioN Tech COVID-19 Vaccine—United States, December 14–23, 2020." *Morbidity and Mortality Weekly Report (MMWR).* https://www.cdc.gov /mmwr/volumes/70/wr/mm7002e1.htm.

Centers for Disease Control and Prevention. n.d. "Local Reactions, Systemic Reactions, Adverse Events, and Serious Adverse Events: Moderna COVID-19 Vaccine." Accessed February 11, 2021. https://www.cdc.gov /vaccines/covid-19/info-by-product/moderna/reactogenicity.html.

Choi, Kristen. 2020. "A Nursing Researcher's Experience in a COVID-19 Vaccine Trial." *JAMA Internal Medicine* 181 (2): 157–58. doi:10.1001 /jamainternmed.2020.7087.

Government of Western Australia Department of Health. n.d. "Comparisons of the Effects of Diseases and the Side Effects of Vaccines." Accessed February 11, 2021. https://ww2.health.wa.gov.au/Articles/A_E/Comparisons-of -the-effects-of-diseases-and-the-side-effects-of-vaccines.

Lewis, Ricki. 2020. "Dr. Paul Offit Talks COVID Vaccines, with JAMA'S Howard Bauchner." *DNA Science.* https://dnascience.plos.org/2020/12/03 /dr-paul-offit-talks-covid-vaccines-with-jamas-howard-bauchner/.

Q4. CAN VACCINES BE PRODUCED FOR ALL DISEASES?

Answer: No. For a vaccine to be developed, the underlying disease, in its natural state, must leave at least some number of patients alive and with an immunity to subsequent exposure to the pathogen. That is, the disease must provoke the immune response that leads to the production of antibodies and T and B cells. As Dr. Anthony Fauci, chief medical advisor to the president, put it, "Natural infection is the mother of all vaccines" (McNeil, 2018).

Many types of diseases do not fit this criterion, such as cancer or heart disease. And many types of infectious diseases mutate so rapidly that vaccines produced to prevent one set of strains won't work against other strains. For example, flu vaccines have to be given every year, because the virus strains that cause the flu mutate while the antibodies produced by the immune system do not. That means that the memory T and B cells produced by the earlier flu strains don't recognize the virus after it has mutated. There is still no reliable vaccine against HIV, the virus that causes AIDS, because the virus not only mutates but also hides in the DNA of immune cells.

In some cases, a vaccine might be technically possible to develop, but not in a cost-effective manner. It would be very expensive to create a vaccine against what we call the "common" cold, for example, because there are actually over 200 rhinoviruses that cause the symptoms we associate with the cold. A vaccine against one rhinovirus would not protect the patient against any other, and colds aren't deadly. Many patients might prefer 200 cases of the cold over their lifetimes to 200 shots.

Vaccine research has historically followed nature's lead, in that the earliest vaccines were developed to prevent the diseases that had the deadliest impact on the population while conveying the longest-lasting immunity to survivors.

The Facts: The terms "vaccine" and "vaccinate" come from research by Edward Jenner (1749–1823) into the use of cowpox, a mild skin disease, to inoculate patients against the deadly and much-feared disease smallpox. Smallpox is caused by two virus variants, or strains, *Variola major* and *Variola minor*. Epidemics caused by *Variola major* were a leading cause of death in Europe and America from the 14th through the 18th centuries. The mortality rate for people who contracted smallpox was approximately 30 percent, and serious side effects among survivors included blindness and disfiguring scars stemming from the disease's most obvious symptom: itchy, fluid-filled pimples known as "pox."

By Jenner's day, there was a well-established practice of inoculating healthy children against smallpox by deliberately infecting them with fluid taken from a child with a mild case of the disease. The children would usually get a similarly mild case of smallpox, exhibiting fever and some number of the pox, but would quickly recover. They were then protected against more serious outbreaks of the disease that they might encounter later in life. By the end of the 18th century, this practice was extended to other vulnerable groups, including soldiers. During the American Revolution, both British and American soldiers were inoculated for smallpox using this method.

Although this practice cut down on mortality and morbidity from smallpox, it was still risky. In some cases, a more virulent strain of the disease would show up in inoculated patients, even if they had been given what appeared to be a mild strain. Some inoculated people became seriously ill and even died. Moreover, patients who were inoculated were as contagious as if they had caught the disease naturally. In order to avoid spreading the infection, they had to be kept isolated until all the pox on their bodies had completely healed. Historians believe that recently inoculated soldiers and members of the Continental Congress were probably responsible for spreading smallpox to civilian populations during the Revolutionary War.

By the 1790s, Jenner was one of a number of physicians looking for a way to preserve the benefits of smallpox inoculation while cutting down on its risks. He decided to investigate a local belief that cowpox, a skin disease frequently contracted by dairymaids and others who worked with cattle, could provide immunity against smallpox. He published his clinical trials, and subsequent follow-up research showed that inoculation with cowpox taken directly from cows could indeed prevent smallpox. For his medical colleagues, Jenner gave cowpox the Latin name Variolae (pox) vaccinae (of cows), and the term "vaccination" was later used to distinguish the material taken from cows from the old inoculation method using smallpox itself. By the end of the 19th century, a related virus, vaccinia, was found to produce the most effective vaccines, and it is still in use today.

Vaccination for smallpox set a high standard for successful immunization practices. Vaccines had to be cost-effective to produce and generate consistently positive results. It had to be successful in protecting the majority of the population and produce much lower mortality and morbidity than even the mildest case of the disease. It also had to cut down on the rate of infection significantly, particularly when combined with other public health measures like quarantine and hospitalization.

Yet, though smallpox vaccination was effective, for most of the 19th century, physicians did not really understand why it worked, because no one had yet established the cause of disease. That changed during the 1860s and 1870s, when scientists first established the germ theory: the theory that a specific disease is caused by a specific microorganism. This theory is the cornerstone of modern medicine, and the research marked the start of the modern sciences of bacteriology (the scientific study of bacteria) and epidemiology (the study of diseases as they occur and spread in different populations). Two famous scientists associated with the germ theory are Robert Koch (1843–1910) in Germany and Louis Pasteur (1822–1895) in France.

Robert Koch began his career as a country doctor with a hobby of scientific investigation into the cause of anthrax, a cattle disease that can also infect people. His success in identifying the microorganism that caused the disease marked the beginning of the scientific study of bacteriology. As the director of the Berlin bacteriological research institute that now bears his name, Koch and his colleagues identified the bacteria associated with over 20 deadly diseases, including anthrax (1877), gonorrhea (1879), tuberculosis (1882), diphtheria (1883), tetanus (1884), plague (1894), dysentery (1898), syphilis (1903), and whooping cough (1906).

Louis Pasteur was a chemist whose early research on bacteriology came from his analysis of wine that had gone bad. He found that the spoiled wine was caused by the presence of microorganisms, each of which had specific biological characteristics. He also found that in many cases, the microorganisms could be destroyed by heating—the process later known as "pasteurization"—or prevented by using sterile techniques for storage. Pasteur, too, established a research institute for the study of microorganisms, focusing on the process for developing what later became known as attenuated vaccines. These types of vaccines use live but weakened versions of the pathogen to produce an immune response.

Live attenuated vaccines are still in use today, though the methods for producing and distributing them are much more sophisticated than they were in the 1890s. Many of the dangerous epidemics of previous centuries, such as smallpox, measles, and yellow fever, are now preventable through live attenuated vaccines.

As microorganisms go, bacteria are comparatively large, and scientists could identify them using 19th-century microscopes and staining techniques. But viruses are much smaller, and the modern field of virology (the study of viruses) only became possible with the development of powerful electron microscopes in the 1930s. In 1953, Jonas Salk (1914–1995) announced that he had successfully tested a vaccine against polio, caused by the poliovirus. Salk had developed an inactivated vaccine—in other words, a vaccine in which the pathogen had been treated so that it was not possible for the vaccinated patient to contract the disease. The modern vaccines for rabies, flu, and hepatitis A are inactivated vaccines.

Some vaccines create an immune response against a toxin (harmful product) manufactured by the pathogen once it is in the body. These are called toxoid vaccines; the most common are the vaccines against diphtheria and tetanus.

Innovative scientific research during the late 20th and early 21st centuries led to a new set of vaccines that target parts of the microorganism rather than the whole pathogen. The vaccine creates the immune response by using fragments of genetic material, such as DNA or mRNA, to generate distinctive structures found on the pathogen. The vaccine against SARS-CoV-2, the virus that causes COVID-19, generates the distinctive protein spike, so that the immune system will recognize it when it encounters the disease. Other diseases for which these kinds of vaccines have been developed are hepatitis B, pneumonia, and meningitis. Often this form of vaccine requires an initial shot plus a booster for full immunity.

As of 2020, there were vaccines approved for 26 diseases in the United States, and full authorization for vaccines against COVID-19 in 2021 brought the number to 27. The World Health Organization estimates that vaccines prevent two to three million deaths every year. However, barriers to developing vaccines exist for some diseases because of the ways they interact with their host organism.

Malaria, one of the oldest of human diseases, illustrates the complications involved in vaccine research. Malaria in humans is caused by four of the *Plasmodium* species of protozoa—a type of single-celled animal—with *Plasmodium falciparum* as the deadliest and most prevalent. There are approximately 200 million cases each year and over 400,000 deaths. It is a serious public health problem in parts of Africa, and children are especially vulnerable to the disease.

Protozoans are among the oldest parasites in human history, and they have evolved a series of ways of preventing the immune system from doing its job. Scientists have identified four distinct stages that the plasmodium goes through once it enters the body, each of which has its own separate antigens. In areas where malaria is endemic, the immune system develops antibodies to all these antigens, but this is not enough to completely prevent later infections. People may therefore contract the disease many times, though generally with milder symptoms over time. *P. faliciparum* also replicate very quickly, leading to mutations that can resist previously formed antibodies. For these reasons, the protozoan has been called a "shape-shifter," creating many challenges in developing an effective vaccine. As of 2019, only one vaccine has been approved for human use; it requires four injections, and its efficacy after all four was only 36 percent. Though research is ongoing to improve the vaccine, the greatest gains against malaria have been made through public health measures to eliminate the mosquitoes that carry it and the development of drugs to treat its symptoms.

Even the most effective vaccines work best when combined with other public health measures. Clean water and effective sanitation prevent the spread of waterborne disease such as cholera, and masks and other social distancing to prevent spread of airborne infectious diseases such as COVID-19.

FURTHER READING

Allen, Arthur. *Vaccine. The Controversial Story of Medicine's Greatest Lifesaver.* 2007. New York: W. W. Norton & Company.

Blevins, Steve, and Michael Bronze. 2010. "Robert Koch and the 'Golden Age' of Bacteriology." *International Journal of Infectious Diseases* 14 (9): e744 c751. https://doi.org/10.1016/j.ijid.2009.12.003.

Duffy, Patrick, and J. Patrick Gorres. 2020. "Malaria Vaccines since 2000: Progress, Priorities, Products." *NPJ Vaccines* 5 (48). https://doi.org/10.1038/s41541-020-0196-3.

Fenn, Elizabeth. 2001 *Pox Americana. The Great Smallpox Epidemic of 1775–1782.* New York: Hill and Wang.

McNeil, Donald. 2018. "Why Don't We Have Vaccines against Everything?" *New York Times.* https://www.nytimes.com/2018/11/19/health/vaccines-poverty.html.

Pardi, N., M. Hogan, F. Porter, et al. 2018. "mRNA Vaccines—A New Era in Vaccinology." *Nature Revies Drug Discovery* 17: 261–79. https://doi .org/10.1038/nrd.2017.243.

Rosner, Lisa. 2017. *Vaccination and Its Critics*. Santa Barbara: ABC-CLIO.

U.S. Department of Health and Human Services. n.d. "Vaccine Types." Accessed February 1, 2021. https://www.vaccines.gov/basics/types.

World Health Organization. n.d. "Vaccines and Immunization." Accessed February 1, 2021. https://www.who.int/health-topics/vaccines-and-immunization #tab=tab_1.

Q5. CAN VACCINES COMPLETELY DESTROY THE DISEASES THEY TARGET?

Answer: No. Vaccines can prevent their targeted diseases from infecting individuals and populations, and they also can prevent those diseases from spreading. But if a pathogen can infect other hosts, or if there is a pool of nonvaccinated individuals in which it can live and reproduce, then the disease will not be completely destroyed. Even a small cluster of cases in a remote area can keep a disease from being eradicated—reduced to zero cases worldwide. Currently, the World Health Organization lists only two diseases as eradicated: smallpox in 1980 and the animal disease rinderpest in 2011.

Vaccines have helped to eliminate a larger number of diseases, which have been reduced to zero cases in a specific area. Polio, for example, has been eliminated in the United States due to its successful vaccination program. The last wild, or naturally occurring, case of polio in the United States was recorded in 1979. A program of polio vaccination has been highly successful in eliminating the disease throughout most of the world. In the 47 countries that make up the African region of the World Health Organization, 220 million children are vaccinated against polio every year, and on August 25, 2020, the region was declared polio-free.

In Afghanistan and Pakistan, the remaining two countries reporting polio cases, public health officials were hopeful that elimination was in sight in 2019, with fewer than 50 cases. Sadly, the infrastructure for polio vaccination, as well as other immunizations, has been disrupted due to the COVID-19 pandemic, and the number of wild polio cases has increased in both countries.

The Facts: The goal of eradicating all diseases goes back to the 19th century, when scientists first developed the methods and expertise necessary to identify microorganisms and develop immunization practices against them. As the next century showed, both eradication and elimination were complex processes, depending on the biology of the microorganism, its perceived threat to human or animal populations, and political and social structures.

By the second half of the 20th century, public health expertise throughout the world had developed a set of criteria to identify diseases that could be eradicated in a cost-effective way. For a disease to be eradicable, it has to be infectious, and we have to have an effective treatment for it. For a vaccine-preventable disease to be eradicated, we have to have a safe, effective vaccine, and we must be able to produce and distribute the vaccine throughout the world.

Another consideration for eradication of a disease has to do with the pathogens that cause it: how many there are, how many variants there are, and how well the vaccine works against them. Yet another consideration is how many hosts carry the disease. If a pathogen only infects one host—people, for example—it is easier to eradicate than if it can be spread by many hosts. For example, a disease like rabies can be almost completely eliminated from humans in a geographical area through rigorous enforcement of rabies vaccination in domestic animals. But there may still be a reservoir of the disease in wild animals in that geographical area.

Other criteria for eradication have to do with the symptoms of the disease: how severe they are and how easy they are to identify. For a disease to be eradicable, public health authorities have to be able to track it, which means there has to be some sort of reliable infrastructure in place for health professionals to report it. This is much more likely to happen when a disease causes severe symptoms, so that infected people have every reason to go to a doctor or clinic. One of the ongoing issues with tracking COVID-19 is that many people who have it have mild symptoms or none at all, so that they have no reason to seek medical treatment. The same reasoning applies to symptoms that can be easily identified, so that both health professionals and members of the community recognize it when they see it. Again, one of the ongoing reporting issues with COVID-19 is that the symptoms resemble those of other respiratory diseases, such as a cold or flu. That makes it hard to track within the population.

The process of tracking a specific disease by public health officials is known as *surveillance*. Two of the most important tools used for surveillance are (1) safe, reliable tests that can accurately determine the existence of a pathogen and (2) contact tracing to track everyone the patient might have infected.

All these criteria have to do with the biology of the pathogen that causes the disease and its impact on the host. Other criteria have to do with the *disease burden*—the social, economic, and political consequences of the disease. Eradication and elimination require a great deal of resources, not only for the production and distribution of vaccines but also for the costs associated with tracking, reporting, and enforcement of public health policies. Marshaling these resources, which may include public health campaigns, quarantine, lockdowns, and social distancing measures as well as immunization, will be more successful in combating a deadly disease that threatens an entire population than in responding to what is perceived as a mild disease threat. This process—the steps taken to prevent the spread of a disease under surveillance—is called containment. Surveillance and containment are the key processes for infectious disease control in the modern world.

The final criteria for a worldwide eradication program is that a disease must have been successfully eliminated in a large geographical area. That effort can serve as a case study to show that eradication efforts are possible. Typically, world health officials look at elimination results in countries that are politically stable with a reliable public health infrastructure. If a disease has not been successfully eliminated in those countries, then it would not be a good candidate for a worldwide eradication campaign.

The smallpox eradication program from 1967 through 1980 shows how all these criteria can be met—but also how hard it can be to meet them. The World Health Organization first set the goal of worldwide smallpox eradication in 1959. By that time, it had already been eliminated in the United States and Europe, and preventing this deadly disease in other parts of the world seemed both technically possible and socially responsible. Smallpox had all the characteristics of an eradicable disease. It is caused by only two pathogens, and both could be prevented with the existing vaccine. Humans also are its only hosts. The symptoms are severe and very visible, and patients are infectious as soon as the symptoms appear. They are therefore very likely to seek treatment, and even if they don't on their own, their symptoms are very obvious to their community. Those factors made surveillance easier than with many diseases. The severity of the disease, and its social and economic impact, provided the political and social environment for enforcing public health policies, including mandatory vaccination.

Unfortunately, for the first effort in the late 1960s, public health officials throughout the world were hampered by vaccines that were hard to transport for a variety of reasons, as well as a complex injection process that was hard to teach to local health care workers. During this same period, however, two technical breakthroughs began to transform smallpox vaccination practices. The first was the application of freeze-drying—first developed by NASA for manned space flight—to smallpox vaccines, making it possible to transport and store the vaccine throughout the world. The second was the invention of the bifurcated needle, which simplified the administration of smallpox vaccines so that it could easily be taught to local vaccinators. Both these innovations contributed to successful smallpox eradication during the 1970s.

Other improvements in vaccination practices revolved around public health professionals' interactions with local communities. In early community public health efforts, doctors working in the field typically would interact with village leaders in identifying households to vaccinate. They vaccinated school-age children who were brought to their attention but were often unaware of younger children or infants in the area who remained unvaccinated. By the 1970s, external doctors and local vaccinators worked closely with families to identify all vulnerable children. They also expanded vaccine administration around an infected individual using what became known as the *ring method*. The ring method involved creating a "ring" of vaccinations around the patient. That meant vaccinating not only family and neighbors but also every single person with whom a smallpox patient had come into contact. If a smallpox patient had been on a bus or gone to the market, public health workers would attempt to track down and vaccinate every person on that bus or in that market.

The deadly impact of smallpox led to additional containment measures that would have been politically or socially difficult to enforce for other, less deadly diseases. In some locations, public health workers offered a reward for information about people who had smallpox. The last known person in the world to have been infected with naturally occurring *Variola major* was three-year-old Rahima Banu from Bhola Island in Bangladesh. Public health authorities heard about the case from an eight-year-old child who received a reward of 250 Taka, about $2.95. Rahima and her family were put under 24-hour house guard, and health care workers carried out a house-to-house vaccination campaign throughout her island. She recovered within a month, and the potential smallpox outbreak was prevented.

The last documented case in which a person was infected with *Variola minor* concerned Ali Maow Maalin, at that point a 23-year-old cook at a hospital in Merca, Somalia. As an adult, he had moved around much more than Rohima and had had many more opportunities to infect others. In addition, Merca is a port city, located near traditionally nomadic groups, and its shifting population made it both likely and dangerous that smallpox could spread outside the area and beyond Somalia. Maalin was isolated and treated, and he worked closely with health officers to identify 161 close contacts and family members. They were also able to set up checkpoints throughout the entrances to the town, maintaining logbooks of all who arrived and departed. They maintained "rash and fever" surveillance and vaccinated all who had not received the smallpox vaccine recently. Maalin recovered, and, once again, a smallpox outbreak was prevented.

Yet for other diseases with similar characteristics, eradication has been more difficult. When the polio eradication campaign was launched in 1988, its promoters were very hopeful that the lessons learned from smallpox could be easily applied. Its biology was as well understood as smallpox, it is caused by only three types of virus, it infects only human hosts, and its vaccine was highly effective. Funding for worldwide eradication was available not only through government agencies but also through philanthropic organizations such as GAVI (the Global Alliance for Vaccines and Immunizations), a partnership of the World Health Organization, the United Nations Children's Fund (UNICEF), the World Bank, the Bill and Melinda Gates Foundation, and other strategic partners. By the year 2000, cases of polio around the world had decreased by 99 percent.

The problem in reaching that last 1 percent lay in part in social and political issues beyond the control of public health officials, such as war and other social disruptions that made it impossible for health care workers to reach vulnerable populations. But part of the problem had to do with the vaccines used in the initial vaccination efforts. The most widely used vaccine for the first 18 years of the polio eradication campaign used a live, attenuated virus, and polio cases emerged that could be directly linked to the vaccine itself. The communities involved became understandably reluctant to be vaccinated. Moreover, misinformation circulated that the needles used in the vaccination process spread HIV, which led to entire communities in Nigeria boycotting the vaccine. From 2016 onward, health care workers used only the form of the vaccine derived from the attenuated virus, and public health officials launched a public education campaign on the value of the vaccine, involving community partners at every level. This direct connection with local communities is a key reason for the successful elimination of polio in Africa.

It is unlikely that COVID-19 will ever be successfully eradicated. The virus mutates too quickly into many variants, the symptoms are often mild or else indistinguishable from other respiratory infections, and the disease burden, once vaccines are generally available, is unlikely to be so severe as to prompt a worldwide eradication campaign. Most likely, the COVID-19 vaccine will be incorporated into yearly immunizations, and mild cases will appear to be yet another version of the common cold.

FURTHER READING

American Museum of Natural History. 2021. *COUNTDOWN TO ZERO: Defeating Disease.* https://www.amnh.org/explore/science-topics/disease-eradication/countdown-to-zero.

Centers for Disease Control and Prevention. n.d. "History of Smallpox." Accessed February 9, 2021. https://www.cdc.gov/smallpox/history/history.html.

Forge, William. 2011. *House on Fire: The Fight to Eradicate Smallpox.* Berkeley, CA: University of California Press.

McVety, Amanda. 2018. *The Rinderpest Campaigns: A Virus, Its Vaccines, and Global Development in the Twentieth Century.* Cambridge: Cambridge University Press.

Roser, Max, Sophie Ochmann, Hannah Behrens, Hannah Ritchie, and Bernadeta Dadonaite. 2016. "Eradication of Diseases." *OurWorldInData.org.* https://ourworldindata.org/eradication-of-diseases.

Rosner, Lisa. 2017. "Global Vaccination Ideals and Realties." *Vaccination and Its Critics.* Santa Barbara: ABC-CLIO, 255–284.

Q6. DO VACCINES EXIST FOR ANIMALS AS WELL AS PEOPLE?

Answer: Yes. Some of the earliest vaccines were developed for animals, and veterinary vaccines play a huge role in keeping household pets and agricultural livestock healthy and free of infectious diseases.

Veterinary vaccines have several purposes. The first is the same as human vaccines: they keep individual animals healthy and prevent their transmitting disease to other animals. The vaccine for canine distemper, for example, protects individual dogs from the infectious and potentially lethal paramyxovirus that causes the disease, and it also prevents its spread to other dogs. As the virus can be spread by direct contact as well as airborne exposure from other dogs, the vaccine is important for keeping the canine population free from this deadly disease.

The second purpose is to prevent the spread of dangerous diseases from animal populations to people. The lyssavirus that causes rabies, for example, is found in the saliva of infected animals, and it can be spread by animal bites to people as well as other animals. Cats, dogs, and people are all vulnerable to rabies, so routine vaccination of cats and dogs helps keep people safe. Anthrax, caused by *Bacillus anthracis*, can also infect people as well as a wide range of livestock and wild animals. Anthrax vaccinations for animals thus also protect people against this potentially dangerous and very infectious disease.

The third purpose of veterinary vaccines is to protect livestock, which is essential for a thriving agricultural economy and the global food supply. Without vaccines, it would be impossible to safely raise and transport the billions of animals that provide meat, fish, poultry, eggs, and dairy products to people worldwide. An infectious disease can run through farm populations like wildfire, decimating both the animal population and the livelihood of people who rely on them. Prior to vaccines, farms large and small were vulnerable to infectious disease. Some farmers saw their entire herd or livestock destroyed as a result of one single outbreak. The global scale of both modern agriculture and modern travel has increased the medical and financial risks associated with infectious diseases.

Chickens, for example, are essential to modern meat production, with an estimated global population of 2.3 billion. Poultry vaccines are a key part of agricultural production and are routinely factored into the cost of poultry farming. Horses are another global commodity, with an estimated 7.3 million in the United States, Argentina, the United Kingdom, France, and Germany. Racing horses may be shipped internationally, and they therefore have the potential to spread infectious disease to local populations. Equine vaccinations keep the animals safe and protect their economic value.

The Facts: Research into animal vaccines was part of the early history of the germ theory. By the mid-19th century, experiments had shown that blood taken from animals who were dying of anthrax could produce the disease when injected into healthy animals. Robert Koch decided to take the research further. He took blood from infected sheep, but instead of injecting it into healthy sheep, he first isolated the cause of the infection— the bacillus—by growing it on an external medium. He allowed it to grow and reproduce for many generations, so that no trace of the original bacillus remained. Then, he injected the bacillus into a healthy animal. He followed this procedure many times, until he had enough evidence to prove that the bacillus caused the disease. His analysis of the life cycle of the anthrax bacillus, published in 1876, became the foundation of modern bacteriological research.

On a personal level, Koch and fellow scientific sleuth Louis Pasteur were bitter rivals, but their experiments followed similar paths. By the 1870s, Pasteur, too, was studying the life cycle of microorganisms, and he had also noted that specific diseases were caused by specific germs. His original interest was in infectious disease of livestock, and his first attempt at creating a vaccine was for chicken cholera, caused by the *Pasteurella multocida* zoonotic bacterium. He tried injecting it into poultry to induce an immune reaction, but he found that too many chickens died. He subsequently experimented with a version that had been stored for some months, leading to a weakened form of the pathogen. That version of the vaccine proved highly effective, and in 1879, Pasteur's chicken cholera vaccine became the first veterinary immunization. Pasteur followed this with a vaccine for anthrax in 1881. His vaccine for rabies, developed for use in dogs, received an unexpected test on a human patient when the mother of a young boy who had been bitten by a rabid dog pleaded with Pasteur to save her son's life. The vaccine, administered under the supervision of a doctor, was successful in saving the boy. By the 1880s, the germ theory was fully established. Over the next 50 years, vaccines were developed for major infectious diseases in animals as well as humans.

Among the most successful animal vaccination efforts was the eradication of rinderpest, an acute, highly infectious disease that infects cattle and other ungulate species, domestic and wild. It is caused by the rinderpest *Morbillivirus*, and throughout history, it spread through long-distance transportation of domestic cattle. In 1889, cattle from India that were carrying the rinderpest virus were shipped to Africa to augment local grazing stock. The resulting epidemic became one of the worst natural disasters ever recorded on the African continent, destroying approximately 90 percent of the cattle population in Africa. The disease rapidly spread to other ungulates as well, killing domestic sheep and goats as well as wild buffalo, giraffes, and wildebeests. The loss of such a huge number of herding and grazing animals led to widespread famine. In regions that depended on herd agriculture for survival, between one and two thirds of the human inhabitants died of starvation and associated diseases.

Koch developed the first vaccine for rinderpest in 1897, but it took another 60 years to develop modern versions that could be easily manufactured and stored for worldwide use. In 1961, Walter Plowright and R. D. Ferris successfully developed a vaccine that could be produced in large quantities, and the later development of freeze-drying techniques allowed it to be used throughout the world. Rinderpest became the focus of public health campaigns in areas where the disease was endemic, such as India and Africa. In 1994, rinderpest became the focus of a World Health Organization eradication campaign, and in 2011 the disease was declared officially eradicated. The campaign is estimated to have cost approximately $3 million, a pittance compared to its economic benefits. It has been estimated, in fact, that eradication of rinderpest increased food production in Africa by $47 billion and in India by $289 billion (FAO, 2010).

The concept of *herd immunity* developed, as the name implies, by vaccination practices associated with remaining healthy livestock herds. The goal of an immunization plan is not only to protect individuals but also to reduce the number of animals that are susceptible to new infections. Once the number of susceptible animals is low enough, the disease will be eliminated in that livestock population. As long as the immunization plan is maintained and no new sources of infection develop, the livestock will continue to be free of disease. For livestock, there may be a reasonable cost-benefit analysis involved in working out an immunization plan, because there is a cost associated with vaccines given to large numbers of animals. If it is possible to save money by vaccinating, for example, only 90 percent of a herd instead of 100 percent, then it may make economic sense for a farmer to do so. The problem arises if the unvaccinated 10 percent end up becoming infected and therefore have to be destroyed. Destroying 10 percent of a herd due to disease is far more expensive than routine vaccination of all the animals.

The concept of herd immunity moved from livestock production to human public health efforts in the 1920s. Today, the term has come to mean the point at which enough people have developed immunity to a pathogen—whether through getting the disease or through vaccination—that the disease is no longer found within that population. But the term has come under criticism when applied to people. For one thing, individual humans are not like individual livestock: it would be completely unethical to have a public health immunization plan that tried to save money by vaccinating some, but not all, susceptible people. For another, people move around at will, rather than being constrained by fences or stockyards used to keep livestock. For those reasons, public health officials prefer the term "population immunity" to "herd immunity."

Use of veterinary vaccines has had additional health benefits for vaccinated animals and the people who rely on them for food and other products. Increased use of vaccines to protect against disease has meant less use of antibiotics to treat those diseases. For example, swine dysentery, a serious disease in pigs, can be treated with antibiotics, but it is more efficient to prevent it with vaccination. This means that farmers and ranchers can use livestock antibiotics more sparingly, and this reduces the likelihood that the animals will develop a resistance to them. Food safety vaccines have also been developed to protect people from foodborne diseases. The vaccines currently available for *E. coli* in cattle and salmonella in chickens do not affect the animals, but they do prevent the outbreaks that would otherwise affect the people who eat them.

In the United States, the production and safety of veterinary vaccines are regulated by the Animal and Plant Health Inspection Service (APHIS) within the U.S. Department of Agriculture (USDA). Laws requiring vaccination of "companion animals"—animals kept as pets—are determined by individual states, but most states require dogs to receive rabies vaccinations in order for their owners to obtain a dog license. Many states require rabies vaccinations for cats as well. The American Animal Hospital Association (AAHA) recommends vaccines against canine distemper and rabies as core vaccines (essential vaccines for all) for dogs, and against rabies, feline panleukopenia, feline herpes virus, feline calicivirus, and feline leukemia virus for cats. Veterinarians may recommend other, noncore vaccinations, depending on the needs of the individual animals.

APHIS determines regulations for vaccines for animals used in agriculture in order to preserve the "health, quality, and marketability of our nation's animals." The agency also promotes national eradication programs, such as the National Tuberculosis Eradication Program, to eliminate bovine tuberculosis (TB) from the cattle population in the United States.

Scientists and government agencies have been able to build on their knowledge of and experience with veterinary vaccines to quickly develop new ones as new disease threats emerge. The equine West Nile virus, for example, was first identified in the United States in August 1999. By August 2001, APHIS had provisionally licensed a new vaccine, and the West Nile virus vaccine has now become one of the core vaccines for horses.

FURTHER READING

American Animal Hospital Association. 2017. "2017 AAHA Canine Vaccination Guidelines." https://www.aaha.org/globalassets/02-guidelines/canine-vaccination/vaccination_recommendation_for_general_practice_table.pdf .

American Association of Equine Practitioners (AAEP). n.d. "Vaccination Guidelines." https://aaep.org/guidelines/vaccination-guidelines.

American Association of Feline Practitioners (AAFP). 2006. "Feline Vaccination Guidelines. Summary: Vaccination in General Practice." https://catvets.com/public/PDFs/PracticeGuidelines/VaccinationGLS-summary.pdf.

American Society for the Prevention of Cruelty to Animals (ASPCA). n.d. "Vaccinations for Your Pet." Accessed January 26, 2021. https://www.aspca.org/pet-care/general-pet-care/vaccinations-your-pet.

Jones, David, and Stefan Helmreich. September 19, 2020. "A History of Herd Immunity." *Lancet* 396 (10254): 810–11. https://doi.org/10.1016/S0140-6736(20)31924-3.

Meeusen, E. N., J. Walker, A. Peters, P. P. Pastoret, and G. Jungersen. 2007. "Current Status of Veterinary Vaccines." *Clinical Microbiology Reviews* 20 (3): 489–510. https://doi.org/10.1128/CMR.00005-07.

Roeder, Peter, Jeffrey Mariner, and Richard Kock. 2013. "Rinderpest: The Veterinary Perspective on Eradication." *Philosophical Transactions of the Royal Society B* 368: 20120139. http://dx.doi.org/10.1098/rstb.2012.0139.

Roth, James. 2011. "Veterinary Vaccines and Their Importance to Animal Health and Public Health." *Procedia in Vaccinology* 5 (2011): 127–36. https://doi.org/10.1016/j.provac.2011.10.009.

Tizard, Ian. 2021. *Vaccines for Veterinarians*. St. Louis: Elsevier, Inc.

United Nations. Food and Agriculture Organization (FAO). 2010. *Lessons Learned from the Eradication of Rinderpest for Controlling Other Transboundary Diseases*. https://www.fao.org/3/i3042e/i3042e.pdf.

United States Department of Agriculture (USDA) Animal and Plant Health Inspection Service (APHIS). 2020. "Animal Disease Information." https://www.aphis.usda.gov/aphis/ourfocus/animalhealth/animal-disease-information.

Q7. ARE NATIONAL AND INTERNATIONAL VACCINATION EFFORTS COST-EFFECTIVE IN SAVING LIVES AND PREVENTING EPIDEMICS?

Answer: Yes. The impact of vaccination, especially childhood vaccination, on national and international health has been carefully studied and assessed. Worldwide, vaccination saves the lives of 6 million people from vaccine-preventable diseases per year. In the United States, it has been estimated that childhood vaccination prevents around 20 million cases of disease and around 42,000 deaths annually. The COVID-19 vaccine has been estimated as saving over 279,000 lives in the United States alone by October 2021 (Greenwood, 2021).

Vaccination for some diseases has been shown to have secondary health benefits. Vaccines may stop the spread of the pathogen entirely, or it may stop the spread of the most virulent strains of the disease, so that even unvaccinated people may get a milder and thus less dangerous form of the disease. Some diseases, like measles, can cause other kinds of unwanted consequences. These include greater vulnerability to respiratory infections, including pneumonia, and the destruction of some of the immune system's previously developed B cells. The latter weakens the immune system by causing a kind of "immunological amnesia": the patient loses some protection against pathogens to which the patient has already been exposed (Rodrigues and Plotkin, 2020). The measles vaccine, therefore, provides protection against more than just measles.

Vaccination also has a clear economic cost benefit or return on investment (ROI), meaning the amount of money saved by investing in vaccine funding. There are two approaches to calculating ROI. The first looks at the cost of illness: the amount of money it costs to vaccinate people compared to the amount of money it would cost to care for those people if they were to become ill or die from the vaccination-preventable disease. Using that measure, researchers have determined that every $1 spent on vaccination programs saves $21 on potential health care costs that have been avoided. The other approach is called a value of statistical life. This calculates all the ways that people who do not die from a vaccine-preventable disease contribute to the economy and society. Using that measure, analysts assert that every $1 spent on vaccination that saves people's lives contributes to $54 in future economic and social benefits generated by those people (GAVI).

The Facts: Since the early 20th century, the introduction of new vaccines has been carefully studied by researchers and governments in order to assess their benefits. In wealthy countries, vaccines are introduced into health care systems as soon as they are developed. In the United States, for example, smallpox vaccination was in widespread use by the turn of the 20th century. Since the 1940s, vaccines were available for diphtheria, pertussis, and tetanus. In the 1950s, the polio vaccine was introduced. In the 1960s, vaccines for measles, mumps, and rubella became available.

By the 21st century, many children in the United States and other wealthy countries only encountered these diseases in novels or movies about historical times. The last case of smallpox in the United States occurred in 1949. There had been an average of 21,000 cases of diphtheria each year in the 1930s, with an average of 1800 deaths. In 1936, there had been as many as 3,000 deaths from diphtheria. But by 2004 diphtheria had been totally eliminated.

Similar vaccination success stories unfolded with other diseases. For example, the United States suffered over 200,000 cases of pertussis each year in the early 1930s, with over 7,500 deaths in 1934 alone. The case load was reduced to around 15,000 by the early 2000s, with 27 deaths in 2004.

Measles, an extremely contagious disease, had averaged over 500,000 cases per year in the 1950s to early 1960s. In 1958 alone, the United States suffered more than 760,000 cases and over 500 deaths from measles. By the early 2000s, there were 55 cases and zero deaths. One study estimated that for children born in the United States in 2009, routine vaccination would lead to a savings in health care costs of $13.5 billion, and $68.8 billion in total societal costs (Zhou et al., 2014).

Many of the studies carried out by the Epidemic Intelligence Service of the Centers for Disease Control (CDC) confirm the value of vaccination. For example, in 1970, an outbreak of 606 cases of measles occurred in the city of Texarkana, located on the border of Texas and Arkansas. Half of the city is in the state of Arkansas, and therefore followed Arkansas laws requiring measles vaccination before entering schools. Only 5 percent of the cases occurred in those districts. The rest of the cases—95 percent— occurred on the Texas side of the city, where there was no statewide vaccination requirement and only 57 percent of the children aged one to nine had been vaccinated.

Another study carried out in the 1960s remains relevant for today because it shows the value of vaccination not just in preventing disease in individual children but also in disrupting and reducing disease transmission in communities. When Rhode Island experienced a measles epidemic in 1965, the state's medical society sponsored a mass vaccination program in which over 30,000 children were vaccinated at 36 clinic sites on a single day—Sunday, January 23, 1966. Follow-up studies over the next two years showed an extremely low incidence of the disease: never, in the state's history, had there been so few measles cases. The study concluded that vaccination had been a timely intervention to stop the disease among the 900,000 inhabitants of the state. These same strategies were used more than a half-century later to disrupt the transmission of COVID-19.

Vaccines can also prevent certain types of cancer. The hepatitis B vaccine has not only protected people from the effects of that disease, but has also decreased the incidence of liver cancer by 50 percent. The human papillomavirus (HPV) vaccine protects against the disease and has also led to a reduction in cervical and other cancers.

Global inequities are the main challenge preventing vaccines from being as cost-effective as they might otherwise be. These inequities follow the main contours of global wealth. At the top end of the vaccine-protected range are children in wealthy countries, such as the United States and many European nations, who may be protected by as many as 13 vaccines against once-deadly childhood infections. These vaccines are administered as part of routine child health care and are generally covered by health insurance or government payments. They ensure that once-dangerous infectious childhood diseases remain things of the past.

In the poorer nations of the world, with low incomes and little health care infrastructure, the vaccination challenges are much greater. As many as 5 percent of children receive no vaccines at all due to lack of availability or expense. In 2019, only 74 percent of children in Africa received the diphtheria-pertussis-tetanus (DPT3) vaccine. Access to this vaccine is often used as a way of measuring access to routine health care, because it requires three separate injections. Although 74 percent is low by world health standards, it nonetheless represents an improvement. In 2000, only 52 percent of children in the region had been vaccinated with DPT3; in 1980, only 5 percent of the region's children had received it.

Even within wealthy countries, there can be great inequities in access to vaccination for rich and poor children. The United States passed the Vaccination Assistance Act in 1962, which empowered the CDC to carry out short-term vaccination programs on an as-needed basis. However, public health officials for most of the 20th century had assumed that routine vaccinations would be carried out by family doctors. By the 1990s, that expectation had been shown to be woefully out of date. As the number of recommended vaccinations increased, the health care insurance available to middle- and upper-class children expanded to cover it. Poor children, who might have little or no health care insurance coverage, might only get the bare minimum of vaccinations necessary to attend public school.

This gap in vaccine equity was widely seen as unfair. "It is unacceptable," stated President Bill Clinton in 1993, "that the United States is the only industrial country that does not guarantee the health of all children. . . . It is ironic that the country that develops and produces the majority of the world's vaccines does not have an effective or affordable mechanism for distributing them to doctors and clinics who treat children" (Rosner, 2017).

Vaccinations were also unacceptably expensive in some cases. This had been clearly shown in the measles outbreak of 1989–91, which resulted in 55,467 cases and 132 deaths. Over 11,000 children were hospitalized as a result of the outbreak, leading to $150 million in direct health care costs. As the children were overwhelmingly from low-income families, the government was responsible for paying that $150 million. At the time, the measles vaccine only cost $24 per shot, so the cost of vaccinating those 55,467 sick children would only have been $1.3 million. The government could thus have saved $148 million by paying for measles vaccination rather than paying for measles treatment.

The Vaccines for Children (VFC) program, established in 1993, provided funds for all recommended vaccinations for low-income children. The Affordable Care Act of 2010 required all health insurance plans to cover recommended vaccinations with no copayment. The results of these efforts, assessed in 2013, were compelling. The VFC was estimated to have protected over 90 percent of children from vaccine-preventable disease. It also was credited with preventing 322 million illnesses, 21 million hospitalizations, and 732,000 premature deaths in the 20-year period from 1994 to 2013. The direct medical cost of VFC to taxpayers was $107 billion. However, analysts emphasized that this cost was actually a bargain, since the cost of providing medical care for all those children if they had not been vaccinated was estimated at $295 billion (Rosner, 2017).

As transportation technology continues to bring different regions of the globe into close contact with one another, vaccination has become both more necessary and more cost-effective. As we have seen with COVID-19, vaccine-preventable diseases are only a suitcase away, and their spread creates not only unacceptably high medical costs, but also severe economic disruption worldwide. The cost of developing, distributing, and administering new vaccines, even if reckoned in the billions of dollars, has come to seem a bargain in comparison.

FURTHER READING

GAVI, the Vaccine Alliance. n.d. "Facts and Figures." Accessed November 30, 2021. https://www.gavi.org/programmes-impact/our-impact/facts-and -figures.

Greenwood, Brian. 2014. "The Contribution of Vaccination to Global Health: Past, Present and Future." *Philosophical Transactions of the Royal Society* B 369 (1645): 20130433. http://dx.doi.org/10.1098/rstb.2013.0433.

Greenwood, Michael. 2021. "U.S. Vaccination Campaign Prevented Up to 279,000 COVID-19 Deaths." *Yale News*. https://news.yale.edu/2021/07/08 /us-vaccination-campaign-prevented-279000-covid-19-deaths.

Hinman, Alan R., Walter A. Orenstein, and Anne Schuchat. 2011. "Vaccine-Preventable Diseases, Immunizations, and the Epidemic Intelligence Service." *American Journal of Epidemiology* 174 (11): S16–S22. https://doi.org/10.1093/aje/kwr306.

Orenstein, Walter, Katherine Seib, Duncan Graham-Rowe, and Seth Berkley. 2014. "Contemporary Vaccine Challenges: Improving Global Health One Shot at a Time." *Science Translational Medicine* 6 (253). https://stm.sciencemag.org/content/6/253/253ps11.

Patenaude, Bryan, and Elizabeth Watts. 2020. "New Evidence Shows Investments in Vaccination Produce Even Greater Returns Than Previously Thought." *Gavi—The Vaccination Alliance*. https://www.gavi.org /vaccineswork/new-evidence-shows-investments-vaccination -produce-even-greater-returns-previously.

Rodrigues, Charlene, and Stanley Plotkin. 2020. "Impact of Vaccines; Health, Economic and Social Perspectives." *Frontiers in Microbiology* 11: 1526. https://doi.org/10.3389/fmicb.2020.01526.

Rosner, Lisa. 2017. "Vaccinating On Time Means Healthier Children, Families, and Communities." *Vaccination and Its Critics.* Santa Barbara: ABC-CLIO, 229–31.

Roush, Sandra, Trudy Murphy, Vaccine-preventable Disease Table Working Group. 2007. "Historical Comparisons of Morbidity and Mortality for Vaccine-Preventable Diseases in the United States." *Journal of the American Medical Association* 298 (18): 2155–63. https://jamanetwork.com/journals/jama/fullarticle/209448.

World Health Organization (WHO). 2020. *Global Vaccine Action Plan. Monitoring, Evaluation, and Accountability. Secretariat Annual Report 2020.* https://www.who.int/publications/i/item/global-vaccine-action-plan-monitoring-evaluation-accountability-secretariat-annual-report-2020.

Zhou, Fanjun, Abigail Shefer, Jay Wenger, Mark Messonnier, Li Yan Wang, Adriana Lopez, Matthew Moore, Trudy V. Murphy, Margaret Cortese, and Lance Rodewald. 2014. "Economic Evaluation of the Routine Childhood Immunization Program in the United States, 2009." *Pediatrics* 133 (4). https://pediatrics.aappublications.org/content/early/2014/02/25/peds.2013-0698.

2

The COVID-19 Pandemic and Vaccine Development

INTRODUCTION

This section answers frequently asked questions about the COVID-19 pandemic and the vaccines that were developed to contain it and protect public health. What was the science and public policy behind the vaccines, and what were the challenges faced in vaccination rollouts? What went into the business decisions on how to ramp up manufacturing? What do we know of the personal stories of adults and teens who participated in clinical trials? What were the ways that governments and philanthropies worked together—or failed to do so—in attempting to bridge the gap between vaccine-rich and vaccine-underserved nations and communities?

From December 2019 through December 2020, people around the globe found themselves catapulted back into a 19th-century disease environment. Many would later describe it as the longest year of their lives, no matter what their age, nationality, or socioeconomic status. The new disease had made its initial appearance in Wuhan, China. It was first identified on December 12, 2019, through a cluster of patients with serious respiratory symptoms. By December 31, 2019, the World Health Organization (WHO) had been notified of a cluster of cases of what looked like pneumonia of "unknown origin"—meaning that doctors and officials did not know what pathogen was responsible for the illnesses or where patients could have encountered it.

By January 7, 2020, Chinese public health authorities had identified the agent as a coronavirus, a type of virus known to cause respiratory symptoms, and they had shared its genetic sequence with global public health authorities. They also identified it as a *novel coronavirus*—one that had never before been found in a human or animal host. By January 21, 2020, Alissa Eckert and Dan Higgins, medical illustrators working for the Centers for Disease Control and Prevention (CDC), had created a visual expression of its genetic identity, including the bright red "spike" protein against a gray-white background. Originally designated as 2019-nCOV, the WHO gave the new disease the official name COVID-19 on February 11, 2020. The virus that causes it was officially called SARS-CoV-2.

In the meantime, the disease appeared outside of China. By January 13, 2020, the first confirmed case appeared in Thailand; by January 15, it was confirmed in Japan. By January 20, the CDC began screening passengers from Wuhan arriving at major U.S. international airports. That same day, a CDC team went to Washington State to investigate a confirmed COVID-19 outbreak. Other countries began experiencing their own, unprecedented outbreaks. By February 23, Italy had become a global COVID-19 hotspot, followed rapidly by comparable outbreaks in other major European countries. Although public health measures were rapidly implemented, the virus had already spread globally via international transportation networks. By March 2020, the disease was confirmed in major U.S. cities. Cruise ships around the world were seriously affected by the disease, with hundreds of cases erupting among passengers and crew.

Public health officials worldwide had long warned that such an outbreak was possible. The SARS epidemic of 2003 and the MERS epidemic of 2012 had made it clear that coronaviruses could be deadly and that they could easily spread among countries and across continents. But both SARS and MERS, though more deadly than COVID-19 on a case-by-case basis, were more easily contained because they were not as contagious. There were 8,439 confirmed cases of SARS and 812 deaths, for a case fatality rate of 9.6 percent, but the disease barely spread outside of China, and no new cases have appeared for many years. Out of the 2,519 confirmed cases of MERS, 866 died, making for a horrifying case fatality rate of 34.3 percent. But again, the disease was comparatively slow to spread, and many of the early deaths were family members and health care workers who came into close contact with early MERS victims. Protective clothing was enough to prevent later fatalities.

COVID-19, while having a much lower case fatality rate, spread incredibly rapidly via casual, person-to-person contact. Any location where people met face to face—schools, restaurants, concerts, weddings, business meetings, political rallies, even doctor's offices—could become a so-called super-spreader event. People aged 65 and older and those with underlying medical conditions were especially vulnerable to serious cases that could prove fatal. By February 2021, more Americans had died of COVID-19 than had died in World War II, the Korean War, and the Vietnam War combined. By August 2021, as the number of cases rose to 46 million and the death toll rose to 750,000, more Americans had died from COVID-19 than from the combination of all those wars plus the Civil War.

Governments around the world imposed stringent measures, including lockdowns and other mandatory public health requirements, to prevent the spread of the disease. But those were never intended to be full solutions. That could only come from a vaccine, and by January 2020, governments from vaccine-producing countries, pharmaceutical companies, and philanthropic organizations had all committed to unprecedented funding for research and development into a vaccine that could tame COVID-19 There were initially 90 vaccine candidates, of which 8 were eventually authorized for emergency use during the pandemic.

The first of the vaccines, developed by Pfizer-BioNTech, was given emergency use authorization for adults by the Food and Drug Administration (FDA) on December 11, 2020. Moderna's vaccine became the second to receive emergency use authorization on December 18, 2020. At first, vaccinations were limited to health care workers, but by January 2020 other groups were added, based on their risk of developing life-threatening symptoms from COVID-19. Those aged 65 and up were eligible first, followed by those aged 18 through 64 who had underlying health conditions such as diabetes or cancer. Scientists calculate that over 140,000 U.S. deaths were averted by the vaccines from January through March 2021. A comparable number of deaths were averted from April through August 2021 by waves of vaccinations.

COVID-19 vaccine development was an amazing success story. As of November 5, 2021, 7.17 billion shots had been given around the world. The vaccines are expected to save the lives of millions of people worldwide, and they gave hope to millions more that even pandemics can be tamed by means of modern science. Yet the story is far from over. The world's wealthiest regions have gotten vaccinated 10 times faster than the poorest ones. Although countries like the United States have enough vaccines to provide full immunization and boosters to every resident, in many low- to middle-income nations, even essential health care personnel are still working without the protection of COVID-19 vaccines. Given this reality, many public health advocates and other observers contend that wealthy nations need to do more to ensure that COVID-19 vaccines, and indeed all vaccines, are equitably and affordably distributed throughout the world.

FURTHER READING

Centers for Disease Control and Prevention. n.d. "CDC Museum Covid-19
    Timeline." Accessed November 4, 2021. https://www.cdc.gov/museum
    /timeline/covid19.html.
Giaimo, Cara. 2020. "The Spiky Blob Seen around the World." *New York
    Times*, April 1, 2020, updated October 9, 2020. https://www.nytimes
    .com/2020/04/01/health/coronavirus-illustration-cdc.html.

Q8. DO WE KNOW WHERE COVID-19 CAME FROM?

Answer: Yes. There are two ways to understand where a disease comes from. The first is its geographic origin, and the second, its evolutionary connection to other diseases. The geographical origin can be very important in trying to prevent a disease from spreading. The evolutionary origin is especially important in helping scientists develop vaccines.

Geographically, we know the first cluster of patients with COVID-19 came from the city of Wuhan, the capital of central China's Hubei province. These early patients were infected with the virus through the city's Huanan seafood and wet animal wholesale market.

Evolutionarily, COVID-19 belongs to the family of coronaviruses, and most scientists believe it is a *zoonotic* disease—that is, a disease that originally affected animals. Under certain conditions, zoonotic diseases can jump over to humans by evolving into a form that can infect them. Because these are, from the human standpoint, new diseases, such "spillover" events can have devastating results, leading to high mortality, high morbidity, and high rates of infection and transmission.

SARS-CoV-2, the virus that causes COVID-19, is called a novel coronavirus because it had not been previous identified. Scientists believe it has been newly introduced to the human population as a disease pathogen. Its closest relatives appear to be two coronavirus strains found in horseshoe bats, which live in many tropical and temperate regions of the world, including Asia. It is not clear at this time whether these strains are the direct evolutionary ancestor of SARS-CoV-2; it may be that both strains evolved from a common ancestor, not yet identified.

SARS-CoV-2 is also an anthroponotic virus, meaning it can be transmitted from people to some animal species. In January 2021, several gorillas at the San Diego Safari Park tested positive for SARS-CoV-2, having caught the disease from a zoo attendant who did not have any symptoms.

In addition, both the United States and other countries reported severe outbreaks of the disease at mink farms. Minks appear to be highly susceptible to SARS-CoV-2, and unfortunately, millions of farm-raised minks have had to be destroyed to prevent further infection. The virus is believed to have spread from people to minks and, in a few instances, from minks to people.

The Facts: People and animals are closely connected through genetics and ecology. It makes sense that they would share diseases as well. As science journalist David Quammen explained in his book *Spillover*, "about sixty percent of all human infectious diseases currently known either cross routinely or have recently crossed between other animals and us" (Quammen, 2012). The good news is that the most dangerous infectious diseases do not jump easily back-and-forth between people and their domesticated pets or livestock. Long association between humans and dogs and cats, as well as cows, horses, pigs, and chickens, means that the immune systems of all those species have adapted to each other. When people do contract diseases from their animals, it is usually through bites—like rabies from unvaccinated dogs—or through ingesting infected animal products.

But sometimes a pathogen that is stable in one animal species—that is, may only cause mild symptoms or none at all—will, through habitat change or other combinations of circumstances, come into contact either directly with people or with domesticated animals. As the pathogen is new to the environment in question, the people and animals do not have any historic immunity to it. The Hendra virus that erupted in Australia in 1994, for example, originated in a bat species and then spread, first to horses and next to people. Since it was identified, 100 horses have died, as have four people exposed to them. A vaccine for horses was introduced in 2012. Like other animal vaccines, it protects both the animals and the humans who care for them.

The human immunodeficiency virus (HIV) strains that cause AIDS, HIV-1, and HIV-2 are also zoonotic. Both strains originated in several species of primates. Scientists have documented mutations in those viruses that suggest at least 12 spillover events from primates to humans during the 20th century. The capacity for mutation that allowed the virus to spread from monkeys to chimpanzees to people also enabled it to infect millions of people worldwide. In the United States, approximately 700,000 people have died from HIV infections since 1981. Worldwide, there have been 3.7 million fatalities.

Although coronaviruses are all zoonotic, they are not all dangerous. Some of them cause mild symptoms that we associate with colds, which suggest that they have been in contact with people for a long time. Coronaviruses were first identified in the 1960s, when technological improvements in electron microscopes and other equipment made it possible to work with viruses in the laboratory. In Great Britain, the Common Cold Research Unit had been set up after World War II to investigate the cause, transmission, and treatment of human "colds." It was understood that what was generally referred to as a single disease, "the common cold," was in fact a cluster of symptoms that could be caused by a number of pathogens.

In 1965, researchers at the Common Cold Unit isolated a virus from a boy with a cold, which they named B814. They found it was "virtually unrelated to any other known virus of the human respiratory tract." Within the next three years, additional viruses with similar structure were identified. In 1968, researchers from several of the teams working in this area wrote to the prominent scientific periodical *Nature*, suggesting that a new category be created for these and other viruses with a similar structure. Although it was not yet possible to identify the characteristic coronavirus spike with the detail we have today, early imaging techniques did show that the viruses had a distinctive appearance, a "characteristic 'fringe' of projections . . . which are rounded or petal shaped . . . recalling the solar corona" (Williams, 2020). For that reason, the scientists suggested, the category should be called coronaviruses.

Researchers soon found that coronaviruses were, in fact, one type of virus that led to cold symptoms. Studies undertaken during the 1960s suggested that approximately 10 percent of all colds were caused by coronaviruses. They did not arouse a lot of research interest or funding, because they did not seem very important. They caused symptoms common to many mild respiratory illnesses, including coughing, runny noses, and sore throats. The illness did not seem to lead to anything worse, and for that reason, it was not considered to be a very high priority for public health or virus research.

That changed in 2002–3, with the outbreak of SARS (severe acute respiratory syndrome), caused by the coronavirus labeled SARS-CoV. The outbreak began in the region in southern China known as the Pearl River Delta. It is one of the wealthiest areas in China, a hub of domestic and international trade and travel. Perhaps most significant for the SARS outbreak, many of the cities in the region had thriving meat markets that specialized in selling meat from wild, rather than farm-raised, animals. Later genomic and field research suggests that SARS-CoV had its origin in local horseshoe bat species. It likely passed to people through infected palm civets, commonly sold for food in the exotic animal markets in the region.

The SARS outbreak began as clusters of what was originally called "atypical" pneumonia, a severe respiratory infection that was resistant to antibiotics, the usual treatment for pneumonia. The virus was both frighteningly dangerous and frighteningly infectious, spreading locally and through international air transportation networks to Beijing, Singapore, Vietnam, Thailand, Taiwan, and even Toronto. Local and global health authorities swung into action, tracing the patients and their contacts and imposing quarantines on those who might carry the infection. The Chinese government also banned the sale of 54 types of animals, including civets, from local meat markets. By the end of the year, the outbreak was contained. Eight thousand ninety-eight people had been infected, and 774 had died. The SARS outbreak was one of the inspirations for the 2011 movie *Contagion*, in which a spillover event at a Chinese restaurant leads to a devastating pandemic.

After the SARS outbreak, public health authorities worldwide breathed a collective sigh of relief that a pandemic had been prevented. They also ramped up research into coronaviruses, since SARS-CoV had shown how deadly they could be. The 2012 outbreak of MERS (Middle East respiratory syndrome) confirmed the potential danger from new coronaviruses.

The coronavirus that causes MERS, labeled MERS-CoV, originated in dromedary camels. The symptoms include the usual ones for respiratory diseases—fever, coughs, and difficulty breathing. It often causes serious illness and has a 35 percent mortality rate. According to WHO, it spread to 27 countries, but the outbreak did not extend to the rest of the world, because the virus is not easily transmitted through person-to-person contact. Generally, human infection seems to require prolonged contact with a sick person. For that reason, most cases spread from sick people to their caregivers, either at home or in a health care setting. Isolating infected people and making sure all caregivers have sterile masks, clothing, and gloves have been effective in preventing the spread of MERS.

By the early 21st century, then, public health officials were aware of the dangers of zoonotic diseases overall, and of coronaviruses in particular. Research carried out as a result of the SARS and MERS outbreaks was to prove enormously helpful in dealing with the much more infectious coronavirus that causes COVID-19.

Although it is possible for people infected with COVID-19 to spread diseases to other animals, the Centers for Disease Control and Prevention does not consider it to be a serious risk for household pets such as cats and dogs. The main risk to domestic animals comes when the humans who look after them become seriously ill and can't take care of them properly.

Public health officials recommend that pet owners who become ill take commonsense precautions. Wherever possible, they should remain isolated from pets as well as family members, and they should make sure that someone is available to care for their animals.

To avoid the spread of infection, pet owners, whether suffering from COVID-19 or not, should make every effort to keep their animals indoors and away from other households. Once again, the basic principles of common sense apply. Pet owners should not put masks on their animals, because animals don't understand the purpose of masks: they will try to rub them off and may even chew and swallow them. People should continue to pet, bathe, and groom their pets in the usual way, as there is no evidence that COVID-19 is transmitted from a pet's skin, fur, or hair. They should not use bleach, hand sanitizer, or cleaning wipes on their pets.

Zoonotic diseases are considered the most likely reservoir for emerging infectious disease outbreaks. Scientists worldwide are engaged in ongoing research programs to develop vaccine candidates as well as treatments.

FURTHER READING

Borell, Brendan. 2018. "Anti-Vaxxers Are Targeting a Vaccine for a Virus Deadlier Than Ebola." *Atlantic*, July 9, 2018. https://www.theatlantic .com/science/archive/2018/07/anti-vaxxers-horses-hendra/559967/.

Centers for Disease Control and Prevention. 2021. "COVID-19 and Animals," February 10, 2021. https://www.cdc.gov/coronavirus/2019-ncov /daily-life-coping/animals.html.

Contagion. 2011. Directed by Stephen Soderbergh. Hollywood: Warner Bros, 2011.

Quammen, David. 2012. *Spillover. Animal Infections and the Next Human Pandemic*. New York: W. W. Norton & Company.

Quammen, David. 2020. "The Virus, the Bats, and Us." *New York Times*, December 11, 2020. https://www.nytimes.com/2020/12/11/opinion/covid -bats.html.

Williams, Shawna. 2020. "A Brief History of Human Coronaviruses." *The Scientist*, June 2, 2020. https://www.the-scientist.com/news-opinion/a-brief -history-of-human-coronaviruses-67600.

Ye Zi-Wei, Shuofeng Yuan, Kit-San Yuen, Sin-Yee Fung, Chi-Ping Chan, and Dong-Yan Jin. 2020. "Zoonotic Origins of Human Coronaviruses." *International Journal of Biological Sciences* 16(10): 1686–97. https:// pubmed.ncbi.nlm.nih.gov/32226286/.

Q9. WERE THE COVID-19 VACCINES ENTIRELY NEW PRODUCTS?

Answer: No. All new scientific breakthroughs rely on previous research. The COVID-19 vaccines were developed out of well-established knowledge about viruses and the vaccines that prevent them. Scientists were able to build on years of tested, trusted research carried out in laboratories, health centers, and field hospitals around the world.

By the 1950s, technological advances had revolutionized the study of viruses. The most notable innovations were the invention of and subsequent improvements to the electron microscope, as well as the development of techniques to grow viruses in cell cultures. By the year 2000, scientists had a whole set of new subjects and technologies to work with. These included discoveries in immunology, the study of the immune system; structural biology, the study of molecular structures and how they fit together inside cells; genetic engineering, the ability to insert pieces of DNA and RNA into cells and have them create new molecular structures; and genome sequencing, the analysis of the precise composition of genetic material. Within the past 10 years, vaccine trials worldwide have been made safer and more effective, so that it is now possible to safely test and administer vaccines during an outbreak.

The SARS outbreak (2003–04) and the MERS outbreak (2013) jump-started the process of vaccine development for coronaviruses. That process slowed down once those outbreaks were contained, but governments and private industry quickly utilized knowledge gained during those earlier events from the outset of the COVID-19 pandemic.

The Facts: From the 1950s onward, research into vaccines for diseases caused by viruses accelerated, leading virologists and historians to refer to the past 70 years as the Golden Age of vaccine development (Plotkin and Plotkin, 2011). From the 1950s through the 1970s, scientists focused on developing viruses by what came to be called classical methods, using attenuated—weakened—viruses. However, they also conducted research using "inactivated viruses," meaning viruses unable to reproduce. (As viruses are not considered to be living organisms, scientists use the word "inactivated" instead of "killed.")

Both attenuated and inactivated virus vaccines required the use of the whole virus to trigger the immune response. In the 1950s, both types of vaccine were developed for polio. In the 1960s, attenuated virus vaccines were developed for measles, mumps, and rubella. In the 1970s, a vaccine for varicella zoster (chickenpox) was developed using attenuated viruses, and a vaccine for Japanese encephalitis was developed using inactivated viruses.

By the 1980s, increased understanding about the immune system, about viruses, and about how to work with genetic material had led to a new approach to vaccines. Through careful research, scientists came to learn that it isn't the whole virus that triggers the immune response but rather a specific molecular structure. More specifically, it isn't the entire coronavirus that triggers the immune system but rather the protein spike. If they could figure out a way to manufacture just the part of the virus that acted as the antigen, they could develop a safer, more effective way of producing the immune response. One of the many genetic engineering tools invented in this period involved using snippets of the virus's DNA to manufacture the desired molecular structures within specific cells. New vaccines for hepatitis B were developed using this technique.

By the 1990s, genetic tools had become sufficiently sophisticated for scientists to look more closely at messenger RNA (mRNA) as a tool for the production of specific biological substances. The mRNA is the genetic material that provides the instructions for the manufacture of proteins, and those proteins carry out key biological roles within the body. As science journalists Damian Garde and Jonathan Saltzman explain, "Researchers understood [mRNA's] role as a recipe book for the body's trillions of cells, but their efforts to expand the menu have come in fits and starts. The concept: By making precise tweaks to synthetic mRNA and injecting people with it, any cell in the body could be transformed into an on-demand drug factory" (Garde and Saltzman, 2020). The problem comes from the immune system itself: when scientists tried to insert the mRNA into a cell culture in the laboratory—the first step in any virus research—it activated the cell's own immune response. The synthetic mRNA was destroyed by the cell it was injected into long before it could become anything like an "on-demand drug factory."

Many researchers worked long and hard on this problem, but Katalin Karikó, a professor at the University of Pennsylvania, has garnered particular praise for her persistence and impact on COVID-19 vaccine research. She worked on the problem of mRNA for 15 years, from 1990 through 2005, before finally achieving a breakthrough technique that would allow the mRNA to slip into the cell under the immune system's wire, where it can transmit instructions that cause the cell to create the antigen protein. Karikó's work and that of her collaborators became the starting point for several start-up companies, including Moderna and BioNTech. By 2010, these and other drug companies, including Pfizer, were at work investigating how to use mRNA techniques to produce a range of pharmaceutical products.

The SARS and MERS epidemics in 2004 and 2012 gave vaccine researchers urgent reasons to ramp up their knowledge of coronaviruses. They had already established that the protein spike acted as an antigen, and teams of scientists around the world poured time, effort, and resources into understanding its structure and behavior. They drew up detailed tables of the types of efficacious vaccines, from those that relied on the classical attenuated and inactivated whole viruses, to those that relied on parts—called subunit vaccines—as well as those that required use of genetic material to create antigens. A particularly promising technique involved creating a strand of DNA wrapped in an inactive adenovirus, a type of virus that usually causes cold symptoms. The researchers, however, had genetically modified the DNA strand so that it no longer caused or spread disease. Once inserted into a cell, the DNA provided instructions for creating the spike protein antigen.

During the SARS outbreak, scientists studied a number of possible vaccine types. One used the inactive whole virus, for example, and another used genetic material. Several vaccines showed promise in both animal trials and early stage human trials. It was not, however, possible to proceed to later trials, because the SARS outbreak was stopped so quickly. Although this was certainly a happy outcome in public health terms, it did mean that there was no way to continue researching vaccines. SARS effectively disappeared as a disease that could be caught naturally, and it was much too dangerous to be given to human subjects under laboratory conditions.

During the MERS outbreak eight years later, those same laboratories took up where they had left off. Though work continued to be done on whole viruses, sometimes with genetically modified features, much of the research was directed toward creating vaccine products that would replicate the antigen qualities of the spike protein, using both mRNA and DNA. A number of laboratories developed potential vaccines that reached the stage of human clinical trials.

Scientists also learned a great deal from the successful development of an Ebola vaccine during an outbreak of that much-feared disease in West Africa in 2013 15. Ebola outbreaks have extremely high mortality, and partly because of that, they tend to flare up and disappear. Essentially, people who contract Ebola often die or become severely ill so quickly that the virus doesn't get an opportunity to jump to other people.

Once an outbreak is over, it is impossible to carry out clinical trials. The World Health Organization (WHO) therefore recognized the importance of testing potential vaccines during the Ebola outbreak. Scientists working for government agencies and private industry used genetic engineering tools to modify the DNA of a livestock virus so that it creates the molecular structure in Ebola that acts as an antigen. After only 20 months, the vaccine, known as rVSV-ZEBOV, was ready for human clinical trials. Human subjects were divided into two groups: those in the first were given the vaccine right away, and those in the second were given the vaccine in three weeks. Of the 2014 subjects in the first group, none developed Ebola, indicating a success rate of 100 percent. In 2019, after additional trials, WHO prequalified the Ebola vaccine, now licensed as Ervebo, for controlled use during outbreaks. Prequalification means that the vaccine meets "WHO standards for quality, safety and efficacy." With the vaccine in place, Ebola has gone from one of the deadliest human infections, with mortality rates from 22 percent to 88 percent, to a "preventable and treatable" disease (WHO, 2019).

By December 2019, when word first spread of yet another coronavirus outbreak (soon to be named COVID-19), scientists were well-prepared to build on the most promising results of the previous 10 years. They had intensively studied two related coronaviruses, and they had a clear understanding of the spike protein and how it latched onto and infected healthy cells in the body. They knew how it triggered the immune response and how antibodies worked on the molecular level to destroy the invading coronavirus and protect healthy cells. They had developed a range of potential candidates for vaccines, and they had carried out trials on the most promising, starting with mice and progressing to primates whose responses most closely matched those of humans. A few had even begun early stage clinical trials on humans. They also had a clear example of the potential for rapid vaccine development during an outbreak, based on the successful timeline for the Ebola vaccine. The COVID-19 vaccines were a great step forward in medicine, but they were not entirely new: they were based on the most successful outcomes of prior research and experience.

FURTHER READING

Butler, Declan, Ewen Callaway, and Erika Check Hayden. 2015. "How Ebola-Vaccine Success Could Reshape Clinical Trial Policy." *Nature*. https://www.nature.com/news/how-ebola-vaccine-success-could-reshape-clinical-trial-policy-1.18121.

Garda, Damian, and Jonathan Saltzman. 2020. "The Story of mRNA: How a Once Dismissed Idea Became a Leading Technology in the COVID Vaccine Race." *Stat*. https://www.statnews.com/2020/11/10/the-story-of-mrna-how-a-once-dismissed-idea-became-a-leading-technology-in-the-covid-vaccine-race/.

Padron-Regalado, Eriko. 2020. "Vaccines for SARS-CoV-2: Lessons from Other Coronavirus Strains." *Infectious Disease Therapies* 9: 255–74. https://www.ncbi.nlm.nih.gov/pmc/articles/PMC7177048/.

Plotkin, Stanley A., and Susan L. Plotkin. 2011. "The Development of Vaccines: How the Past Led to the Future." *Nature Reviews Microbiology* 9: 889–93. https://www.nature.com/articles/nrmicro2668.

World Health Organization. 2019. "WHO Prequalifies Ebola Vaccine, Paving the Way for Its Use in High-Risk Countries." https://www.who.int /news/item/12-11-2019-who-prequalifies-ebola-vaccine-paving -the-way-for-its-use-in-high-risk-countries.

Q10. DID THE SEVERE IMPACT OF COVID-19 ON GLOBAL HEALTH SPEED UP THE PROCESS FOR DEVELOPING VACCINES?

Answer: Yes. COVID-19 was recognized as a world health crisis right away. The World Health Organization (WHO) and national governments worldwide adapted existing emergency procedures to speed up the process for developing COVID-19 vaccines.

Although the COVID-19 vaccines were developed rapidly, they were tested rigorously, according to the same safety protocols employed for all other vaccines. In fact, because of global concerns about safety, the vaccines were developed with heightened attention, and with much more information publicly available about the process than usual. The increased focus on safety continued during the vaccine rollout, with health officials worldwide sharing data and keeping track of side effects and adverse reactions.

Three conditions led to the safe, effective, and rapid manufacture of COVID-19 vaccines. The first two were discussed in the previous section: (1) existing scientific knowledge about viruses and how to work with them to create new vaccines; and (2) the flood of research into coronaviruses prompted by the SARS and MERS outbreaks that led to preclinical and clinical trials. The third factor that helped drive the quick development of effective COVID-19 vaccines was the worldwide spread of COVID-19 itself. Researchers were thus able to recruit thousands of volunteers for rigorous, double-blind clinical trials and ensure that the results of those trials could be applied to the larger population.

The Facts: For most vaccines, development is a long process, taking between 10 and 15 years. It was possible to jump-start the process for COVID-19 vaccines because a great deal of the preliminary research had already been carried out. When confronted by the pandemic, scientists were able to draw on 60 years of research into coronaviruses, 30 years of research into using fragments of viruses as antigens, and 20 years of research into developing vaccine products from those fragments. They were also able to draw on the example of rapid-fire development during the 2013–15 outbreak of Ebola in West Africa, when an international collaboration of scientists, funders, and government agencies worked together to produce an effective vaccine in just 20 months. This previous work made it possible to produce several safe, effective vaccines against COVID-19 in approximately one year.

As soon as the dangers of COVID-19 were made public, scientists with a track record of vaccine research began gearing up to produce a vaccine. Sponsors of vaccine research range from government laboratories to universities to private industry, and they both compete and collaborate with one another. To coordinate the efforts in the United States, the federal government created Operation Warp Speed, a collaboration between the Department of Health and Human Services (HHS), which includes the Food and Drug Administration (FDA) and the Centers for Disease Control and Prevention (CDC), and the Department of Defense (DOD). Operation Warp Speed disbursed $13 billion in federal funding for research, development, testing, and distribution of COVID-19 vaccines, $10 billion of which came from the CARES (Coronavirus Aid, Relief, and. Economic Security) Act. In January 2021, when the Trump administration gave way to the presidency of Joe Biden, the name Operation Warp Speed was retired and its operations were transferred to the White House COVID-19 Response Team.

As government officials crafted the process to facilitate vaccine development, they took seriously the lessons learned from previous attempts at vaccine development during an outbreak. Their first commitment was to maintain the high standards of efficacy and safety that would be part of any vaccine review process. The HHS therefore made the determination that the FDA would retain its role as independent regulator of vaccine products. Career scientists within the agency and external experts convened as part of its advisory body, the Center for Biologics Evaluation and Research's (CBER) Vaccines and Related Biological Products Advisory Committee (VRBPAC), were held to the usual rigorous standards to avoid conflict of interest or any suspicion of political bias.

In order to understand how the development of COVID-19 vaccines could proceed so rapidly without loss of safety and efficacy, we can review the usual process for vaccine development when there isn't a pandemic. Before the formal process of vaccine approval even gets started, there must be years of scientific research in laboratories all over the world to provide a clear understanding of the pathogen and how it enters and affects the body. In the 21st century, these studies have focused on decoding the genome, or the genetic code, of the organism that causes the disease, as well as the life cycle of the microorganism and the specific molecular behaviors that allow it to attack its host. Scientists also study the body's response to the pathogen, including the specific trigger that activates the immune response, and the precise structure of the antibodies and the killer T cells that combat it.

This basic research has been especially dramatic in the study of viruses, because they consist of strands of DNA or RNA wrapped in a protein coat. The application of DNA sequencing, a staple of genetics research since the 1970s, has enabled virologists to make enormous strides in the understanding of disease-causing viruses. A new field of science, computational biology—computers applied to biological research—has made it possible to identify and sequence viruses in real time during outbreaks and to track variants as they develop.

Once a disease-producing microorganism is well understood, government, university, and industry laboratories are ready to start the formal process for developing a vaccine. In the United States, all vaccines must be licensed by the FDA, and other countries have similar regulatory bodies. There are clear guidelines that vaccine manufacturers must follow, and the whole process is carefully monitored.

The first phase of vaccine development is known as the exploratory phase. It consists of developing and testing biological substances to see if one will act as an antigen to trigger the immune response. Under nonpandemic conditions, this can take from two to four years. Historically, vaccines have been weakened or inactivated versions of the original pathogen. Since the 1990s, though, scientists have applied their knowledge of molecular structures to create new kinds of vaccines, which mimic only the part of the virus that triggers the immune response. Researchers must show that they can create the substance under laboratory conditions, and that it can be stored in a stable condition, in order to move on to the next stage of the process.

During the next, preclinical stage, sometimes known as the animal trials stage, researchers work with tissue cultures and with animals to show that the biological substance can, in fact, produce an immune response. The process is carefully controlled to provide information about dosage, about how effective the substance is in protecting live organisms against the disease, and about any adverse reactions. This stage can last for one to two years. It is often the make-or-break stage, because most of the substances developed do not, in fact, convey immunity.

If the substance—known at this stage as the candidate vaccine—passes successfully through the preclinical stage, then it can, if approved, move into clinical trials on human subjects. In the United States, any companies wishing to carry out the clinical trial stage must apply to the FDA for an Investigational New Drug (IND). All applications are reviewed by a clinical review board. This approval process usually takes 30 days. The sponsor must give precise information on the candidate vaccine, including the development process and all information gathered from the preclinical trials. The sponsor must also provide precise information on the plan for clinical trials, including information on efficacy and safety.

If the IND is approved, the candidate vaccine can move into clinical trials on human subjects. Phase 1 trials ordinarily involve 20–80 subjects and last about one year. All subjects must volunteer for the trials, and they must be informed of the risks of the trials. Their health and well-being must be closely monitored. Both the candidate vaccine and placebos are administered, but at this stage, the trials do not have to be blinded: that is, both patients and health care professionals may know who has the vaccine and who has the placebo. The goals of Phase 1 trials are to make sure that the candidate vaccine does, in fact, produce an immune response in the form of antibodies, and that it does not cause any serious adverse effects. This phase also begins to address logistics issues, such as dosage, manufacturing constraints, and storage requirements.

If the candidate vaccine fulfills the expectations of Phase 1, it moves on to Phase 2, which includes several hundred adult test subjects and ordinarily lasts about a year. This time, the studies are randomized and double-blinded, which means that neither the subjects nor the health care professionals know who is getting the placebo and who is getting the vaccine. Researchers may try to include subjects who are especially at risk for the disease. The goals are to rigorously test the differences between the responses of those who got the vaccine and those who got the placebo. Researchers look for evidence that the vaccine candidate is efficacious. Evidence for this may come from lab testing for antibodies, and it may also come from data showing that subjects in the vaccine group caught the disease in lower numbers than those in the placebo group. Researchers also look for evidence that it is safe, and they carefully monitor any reports from subjects about side effects.

If the candidate vaccine has made it through the previous stages, it is ready for Phase 3, which consists of large clinical trials, usually between 1,000 and 10,000 adults. This is a full-scale version of the double-blind studies in Phase 2, expanded to ensure that even rare adverse effects will show up. They can take as long as three years, in part because there has to be time for subjects to be exposed to the disease. That may mean that the trials have to take place at multiple sites, and even multiple countries, to ensure that there are enough people affected by the disease. The key questions for Phase 3 are as follows: Does the data show that the vaccine prevents the disease in the field, that is, are subjects who received the vaccine catching the disease in significantly smaller numbers than those who received the placebo? Does the lab testing for antibodies support that evidence? How long do the antibodies last? Are there side effects? If so, what is the range and variety of side effects? Can the vaccine be successfully manufactured within a reasonable time frame? What are the requirements for storage and distribution?

Only after these trials have been completed successfully can a sponsor submit a Biologics License Application to the FDA. The application goes through rigorous review by career scientists within the agency, and by external experts. If the license is approved, the company can then begin manufacture and distribution of the licensed vaccine. Both the company that develops the vaccine, and the FDA, continues to monitor it for safety and efficacy.

This is usually a careful and slow-moving process, best suited to an ordinary healthcare environment, not a national or international health crisis. Under emergency conditions, the FDA can set up emergency procedures to speed up development and distribution of vaccines, treatments, and medical supplies. They also issue an Emergency Use Authorization (EUA) for medical materials that have passed rigorous standards for safety and efficacy.

During the COVID-19 pandemic, all stakeholders in vaccine research worked hard to make the process as efficient as possible, while maintaining the usual high safety standards. Government officials awarded funding to potential vaccine sponsors that had specific characteristics. First, they had to already have completed preclinical and clinical trials, with convincing evidence that their candidate vaccines would be safe and effective. Second, they had to provide convincing evidence that they would be in position to carry out large-scale Phase 3 trials from July 2020 through November 2020, with convincing evidence of safety and efficacy by the first half of 2021. Third, they had to provide convincing evidence that they already had in place the facilities to manufacture and distribute the vaccines. That meant that any special requirements, such as extra-cold refrigeration, had to be designed and tested by the time successful clinical trials had been concluded.

To further speed up the process, each company was authorized to develop one type of vaccine, and each was expected to devote the majority of their resources to that vaccine. Companies were, in effect, being asked to put all their eggs in one basket, in order to make most efficient use of their resources. Both Pfizer and Moderna chose mRNA technology, while Johnson & Johnson and AstraZeneca chose DNA wrapped in an adenovirus. This process ensured that companies were concentrating on creating the vaccine product they knew and understood most, rather than trying to create a whole array of products that might spread their resources too thin.

The main technique used to speed up the development timeline was staggering the separate clinical stages, rather than running them in sequence. This technique had been found to be very effective during the Ebola vaccine trials in 2014–15. During nonoutbreak conditions, a company might complete Phase 1 trials, write a report over several weeks or even months, and then leave additional time to consult with the FDA before beginning Phase 2. The same would be true on completion of Phase 2 trials. If the disease for which the vaccination was being developed was not very prevalent, Phase 3 trials might take months or years until a sufficient number of vulnerable subjects could be found.

Under outbreak conditions, however, companies had found ways to cut the timeline considerably. Once they had evidence from preclinical and Phase 1 studies to show a vaccine was safe and to indicate an effective dose, they could begin Phase 2 and Phase 3 trials. Moderna, for example, had begun Phase 1 trials in March 2020; the trial ran through November 2021. Phase 2 ran from May 2020 through August 2021. Phase 3 began in July 2020 and ran through October 2022. By December 2020, as the first doses of their vaccine for adults was approved, scientists had begun work on Phase 2 and 3 clinical trials for adolescents aged 12–18.

By December 2020, both Pfizer and Moderna had developed candidate vaccines that met the FDA gold standard for safety and efficacy. As their trials had not yet been completed, they could not take the step of completing a Biologics License Application, which grants approval from the FDA to manufacture a biological product. Instead, they applied for an EUA, which is, as the name implies, an authorization for a product to be used due to a national emergency. An EUA is only granted to a product that meets rigorous FDA review, and it lasts only during the federally declared emergency.

In order to receive an EUA for their COVID-19 vaccines, companies had to provide scientific data to clearly demonstrate that the benefits of the vaccine clearly outweighed the risks for its targeted patient population. They had to provide evidence that they could consistently manufacture millions of doses of a high-quality vaccine. They had to provide "clear and compelling safety and efficacy data" from Phase 3 clinical trials to show that the benefits of the vaccine to "millions of individuals" from a range of ages and ethnicities outweighed the risks. Finally, they had to provide plans for continued study and monitoring of the vaccines through ongoing clinical trials and through its use under emergency authorization (Fink, 2020).

The COVID-19 vaccines that received EUA have been administered to millions of U.S. residents, and they have confirmed the clinical results of their safety and efficacy. The Pfizer-BioNTech COVID-19 vaccine received full FDA approval for its Biologics License Application on August 23, 2021. Moderna and Johnson & Johnson have submitted their Biologics License Application for their COVID-19 vaccines as well, and FDA approval is expected by late 2021 or early 2022.

FURTHER READING

Centers for Disease Control and Prevention. n.d. "Vaccine Testing and the Approval Process." Accessed March 19, 2021. https://www.cdc.gov/vaccines/basics/test-approve.html.

Fink, Doran. 2020. "Emergency Use Authorization Overview and Considerations for COVID-19 Vaccines." *Food and Drug Administration*. https://www.fda.gov/media/144329/download.

Food and Drug Administration. n.d. "Emergency Use Authorization for Vaccines Explained." Accessed March 19, 2020. https://www.fda.gov/vaccines-blood-biologics/vaccines/emergency-use-authorization-vaccines-explained.

U.S. Government Accountability Office. 2021. "Operation Warp Speed. Accelerated COVID-19 Vaccine Development Status and Efforts to Address Manufacturing Challenges." GAO-21-319, February 2021. https://www.gao.gov/products/gao-21-319.

Q11. WAS IT CHALLENGING FOR COMPANIES TO CREATE THE COVID-19 VACCINES SO QUICKLY?

Answer: Yes. Even biomedical companies that had been working on vaccines for decades found it challenging to ramp up research, development, and distribution to be able to deliver a vaccine in approximately one year. In order to promote confidence in the new vaccines, companies were transparent about the hurdles they faced and how they overcame them. As a result, we have a great deal of information about how to manufacture vaccines rapidly and how to distribute them efficiently in times of need.

As discussed in Q8 and Q9, three factors helped create the environment that made rapid development of COVID-19 vaccines possible. Research scientists could base their work on many years of advance research, companies could count on government funding for research and development (as well as government contracts once the vaccines were authorized), and the disease was widespread enough to quickly obtain significant results in clinical trials. Even so, companies had to evolve new business models and practices in order to make their targeted deadlines and ensure safe, effective vaccines would be available and accessible to billions of people worldwide.

The Facts: The main challenge reported by everyone involved in the COVID-19 vaccine development process was the compressed timeline. In an ordinary development process, activities follow a set process: first, vaccine research and development; next, testing; then regulatory approval; then manufacturing; and then distribution. The timelines are set by previous experience in vaccine development and manufacturing. It is really much the same process as seen in any other manufactured product. For example, when automobile companies design a new car model, designers and engineers review their existing models and decide how to change, upgrade, and improve it, based on the automotive market and the manufacturing priorities of the particular car company. Once the model is designed, it is tested to ensure it meets all regulatory standards. Once those tests are reviewed and approved, the cars can be manufactured at the company's already existing factories. Once the specified number has been produced, the cars can be shipped to new car dealerships. The number of cars and the timing of sales can be reasonably predicted from previous years, and so the production and distribution schedule changes very little from previous years.

The same is true with many vaccines. It is reasonably predictable how many children will be born each year, and so it is part of the standard business model of pharmaceutical companies to manufacture and distribute the required number of childhood vaccines in a given year. The same is true of seasonal flu patterns; pharmaceutical companies can work with previous years' data in following an orderly process for ensuring that enough flu vaccines are available each fall.

But companies working on the COVID-19 vaccines did not have the luxury of following an established procedure. Instead, they had to look for ways to develop and test multiple candidate vaccines while upgrading or, in some cases, building entirely new manufacturing plants and distribution networks. They also had to maintain frequent—in some cases, daily—contact with regulatory agencies to make sure they were meeting the most rigorous standards for safety as well as efficacy. The steps they took have become case studies in business and health care innovation.

Since the first COVID-19 vaccine to receive Emergency Use Authorization came from a collaboration between the U.S. pharmaceutical company Pfizer and the German mRNA company BioNTech, their process has received the most attention. We can follow the timeline of both companies from January 2020 through December 2020 to see how they coped with challenges.

By January 2020, it was clear to pharmaceutical companies that, horrible as the prospect of a global COVID-19 pandemic was, it also represented a major opportunity for vaccine research and development. BioNTech, located in Mainz, Germany, was a comparatively small company with only about 1,000 employees, but its core research centered on working with mRNA to create new biological products. The company had developed proprietary software that could take the genetic information for a coronavirus and provide instructions on how to mimic the distinctive protein spike. On January 25, 2020, the company's chief executive, Ugur Sahin, plugged COVID-19 information into the software and generated 10 possible candidate vaccines. When he turned the problem over to company research scientists, they generated another 10. That gave them the blueprints for 20 potential vaccines, each of which would need to be manufactured in small doses and tested first on laboratory animals and then, if successful, on people.

As a small company, BioNTech had been focused on the research and development side of mRNA vaccines. They didn't have the resources necessary for clinical trials or manufacturing. However, they had previously partnered with Pfizer, a well-established pharmaceutical company with a long track record in successful vaccines and over 78,000 employees, to develop a flu vaccine using mRNA technology. On March 1, 2020, Sahin discussed collaboration with Dr. Kathryn Jansen, Pfizer's director of vaccine research. "This is a disaster, and it's getting worse," Dr. Jansen told Dr. Sahin. "Happy to work with you" (Hopkins, 2020).

Pfizer's chief executive, Albert Bourla, gave his approval a week later. Bourla, Jansen, and other top executives at Pfizer held virtual meetings twice a week to make sure they stayed on top of the leadership process. From the first, Bourla insisted on an October 2020 delivery date for the vaccines. Though the company did not quite make that deadline, even those who pushed back against what they considered to be unrealistic expectations gave Bourla credit for the successful delivery of safe, effective vaccines in record time.

Also in March 2020, Mike McDermott, head of Pfizer's manufacturing team, started the process for actually producing the vaccines. Ordinarily this would wait until the company had decided upon a specific vaccine candidate, so all the manufacturing requirements, such as dosage and storage, would be tailored to that candidate. But Pfizer did not, at that point, have any facilities for manufacturing mRNA vaccines: they would have to be built from scratch—and the sooner, the better. A plant in Massachusetts was set up to make the mRNA, and another was established in St. Louis, Missouri, to provide the raw materials needed. In order to avoid any delays, Pfizer decided to use their own money to build and design the necessary equipment, rather than waiting for government funding to come through. That decision, while costly, may have saved them three vital weeks in manufacturing time.

By April 2020, BioNTech and Pfizer scientists, working together, had eliminated 16 of the 20 candidate vaccines. They had carried out preliminary animal trials on the remaining four using monkeys, and they had been sending data updates to the Food and Drug Administration (FDA). As the animal trials indicated that there were no serious adverse effects to any of the four candidate vaccines, they received approval to try them out on small groups of human volunteers. In the trials for two of the potential vaccines, some subjects experienced chills and fevers, and so those were discarded. That left two potential vaccines, and human trials were scheduled to continue through July 23. Pfizer told the FDA that they would inform them of the results on July 24.

Also in April 2020, Pfizer purchased and began building formulation machines, which are key components of the mRNA manufacturing process. These machines take the mRNA and put it in the lipid coat that allows it to enter cells and begin its work of manufacturing spike antigens. The company started planning for the production process, which includes one week to make the mRNA components, and then two weeks to test them. Around the same time, Pfizer's manufacturing division began producing storage containers that could store the vaccine at cold temperatures. The precise range of temperature the vaccines might need wasn't known, because the final vaccine itself wasn't yet known. They therefore decided to go with subarctic temperatures, to make sure the vaccine would be stored in the safest possible way. To test the storage process, they put the containers on cargo ships to Dubai and Africa and also shipped them to Pfizer employees' houses. Since there were still two viable candidates at this stage, the company had to make sure that it had the capability to produce and distribute whichever one the scientific team finally chose.

Producing the vaccine was actually a two-stage process. The first stage involved producing enough vaccines for the clinical trials. The second involved producing enough for actual distribution to the public. Due to the time constraints, the manufacturing team had to plan for both simultaneously. That process received an additional challenge when, on June 30, 2021, the FDA decided the Phase 3 clinical trials should include 30,000 subjects, rather than the original 8,000. With Pfizer clinical trials scheduled to begin in July, the manufacturing team had to ramp up production for the additional 22,000 doses, again without knowing which candidate vaccine would ultimately be chosen.

On July 23, 2020, the Pfizer vaccine research team decided on the second of the two vaccine candidates, and on July 24, 2020, it provided the required data to the FDA. Recruiting volunteer subjects for the trials was already in process, and on July 27, the first four volunteers received injections. The researchers planning the trials tried to schedule them in known COVID-19 hot spots, to make sure that those enrolled would have plenty of natural exposure to the disease. They ran into an unexpected snag, however, when fewer subjects than expected in the placebo group tested positive for COVID-19. Pfizer scientists were puzzled, but assumed that it had to do with behavior among all the volunteers, who were urged to wear face masks and follow social distancing guidelines. Moreover, by the end of the summer, infections rates were not as high in the locations where the original clinical trials had been set up. Pfizer scientists had to switch their locations to emerging hotspots in other parts of the world. By early November, preliminary results had shown that the vaccine, delivered in two doses, was more than 90 percent effective.

Once again, Pfizer's manufacturing team had been working parallel to the scientific team. By mid-August 2020, the company's factory in Belgium had begun producing the vaccine, and by the end of September, it had 1.5 million doses ready to ship as soon as it was authorized in any country. As vaccine scientists worked on the clinical trials in September and October, engineers installed and tested the machines necessary for full-scale industrial production. Although they were not able to produce the 100 million doses by October that Bourla had wished, they had 50 million ready for distribution by the time the FDA granted Emergency Use Authorization for the Pfizer-BioNTech COVID-19 vaccine on December 11, 2020.

As Bourla put it, "I always try to shoot for the stars, because I know that even if you miss it, you will land somewhere in the moon," he said. "But right now it looks like we landed, more or less, in the stars" (Hopkins, 2020).

FURTHER READING

Centers for Disease Control and Prevention. 2021. "Information about the Pfizer-BioNTech COVID-19 Vaccine." https://www.cdc.gov/coronavirus /2019-ncov/vaccines/different-vaccines/Pfizer-BioNTech.html.

Food and Drug Administration. n.d. "Pfizer-BioNTech COVID-19 Vaccine."
    Accessed March 26, 2021. https://www.fda.gov/emergency-preparedness
    -and-response/coronavirus-disease-2019-covid-19/pfizer-biontech
    -covid-19-vaccine.
Harper, Matthew. 2020. "In the Race for a Covid-19 Vaccine, Pfizer Turns
    to a Scientist with a History of Defying Skeptics—And Getting Results."
    Stat. https://www.statnews.com/2020/08/24/pfizer-edge-in-the-race-for-a
    -covid-19-vaccine-could-be-a-scientist-with-two-best-sellers-to-her
    -credit/.
Hopkins, Jared. 2020. "How Pfizer Delivered a Covid Vaccine in Record
    Time: Crazy Deadlines, a Pushy CEO." *Wall Street Journal.* https://www
    .wsj.com/articles/how-pfizer-delivered-a-covid-vaccine-in-record
    -time-crazy-deadlines-a-pushy-ceo-11607740483.

Q12. DID RAPID DISTRIBUTION OF COVID-19 VACCINES IN THE UNITED STATES POSE MAJOR CHALLENGES?

Answer: Yes. Developing and distributing the vaccines during an ongoing pandemic created numerous challenges for federal, state, tribal, territorial, and local public health officials. A large part of the problem stemmed from the fact that coordination between federal officials and local government agencies was already strained by COVID-19 relief efforts during the first six months of the pandemic.

In addition, the ongoing federal efforts to develop the vaccines gave little initial consideration to how they would be administered. Instead, distribution was left up to state, tribal, territorial, and local officials, who had very limited information on either the time frame for delivery or the number of doses that would be allocated to them. Many reports issued by the U.S. Government Accountability Office (GAO) highlight how this lack of information from federal authorities led to costly and time-consuming delays in vaccine rollout and delivery.

Other complications with vaccine distribution cropped up as well. Once vaccines were available, they were first allocated for the most vulnerable— people over 65 or those with illnesses that made them especially at risk from severe cases of COVID-19. However, early vaccine registration systems required use of computers or smart phones, often an inappropriate technology for the intended elderly age group. Another complication was that that early vaccination outreach efforts followed the same racial and income disparities as the American health care system, so that Black, Hispanic, and

Native American patients had less access to the vaccine than their white counterparts.

The Facts: The vaccines used during the COVID-19 pandemic were developed and rigorously tested. The Pfizer-BioNTech vaccine received Emergency Use Authorization (EUA) on December 11, 2020, and the Moderna vaccine received its authorization on December 18, 2020. These vaccines gave hope to millions, but the EUA was only the first step. The next six months revealed many bumps in the road for the vaccine rollout. State agencies; public health officials; and nurses, doctors, and other medical personnel did their best throughout to meet and circumvent each challenge as it arose.

The first set of challenges to distribution had come up during the process of manufacturing the new vaccines on the scale needed to end the pandemic. One problem was locating and preparing manufacturing facilities for production of the new vaccine. Pharmaceutical companies, like other businesses involved in manufacturing, don't like to see their plants sitting idle. For that reason, they carefully match manufacturing activity to anticipated need. As a result, neither Pfizer nor Moderna had much in the way of free manufacturing space to produce the new vaccines.

Moreover, under ordinary circumstances, vaccine manufacturing increases gradually, as a new vaccine comes on the market for a specific disease. During the COVID-19 pandemic, however, companies had to locate, build, and equip entirely new facilities from the ground up, in a matter of months. They were particularly hard pressed in manufacturing sterile storage containers—vials and syringes—that would allow for safe and convenient distribution to health care facilities. These had to be manufactured to the precise requirements of the new vaccines, and those requirements had only been firmly established a few months before distribution was scheduled to start. The result was a series of manufacturing bottlenecks that were not fully worked out until several months after the EUAs had been approved.

Another issue was the gaps in manufacturing supply chains caused by the pandemic's worldwide disruptions to production and shipment of medical supplies. From chemicals to containers, reagents to reactor bags, materials that would ordinarily take a week to arrive were delayed from one to three months.

Even more disruptive was the severe shortage in trained personnel, including people who would ordinarily fill the role of project managers. Vaccine development project managers are specialized positions within pharmaceutical companies. Under ordinary circumstances, personnel necessary to manufacture and distribute new vaccines would be hired as part of the same gradual process as setting up the manufacturing plant. Under pandemic conditions, it became much more difficult to hire knowledgeable, experienced staff.

A serious challenge to effective distribution of the vaccines came from the disconnect between the officials appointed by President Donald Trump to oversee the development of vaccines and the nonfederal jurisdictions whose job it was to distribute them. These included all 50 states, 16 territories, Tribal nations, the District of Columbia, and cities with their own public health agencies: Chicago, Houston, New York City, Philadelphia, and San Antonio. Having taken steps to produce the vaccine, federal officials initially left it up to the local jurisdiction to distribute it, with very little federal-to-local planning or communication.

In September 2020, the GAO called for a clear plan for distribution, one that followed best practices in project management and provided "timely, clear, and consistent" information to all the jurisdictions responsible, so that they could plan for the vaccine rollout (GAO-21-443 September 2020, 4). As the GAO noted in January 2021, however, their interviews with "state, territorial, and local health officials and health care providers" showed that federal agencies did not follow best practices. According to the GAO report, local administrators had to cope with "competing priorities with limited resources and lack of information needed for on-the-ground planning for vaccine administration" (GAO-21-443 September 2020, 32).

Lack of adequate guidance from the Trump administration created problems for those "on the ground." Federal agencies shipped vaccines across the country according to a formula based on population. However, public health officials on the receiving end were not given clear information on the number of doses that would be shipped or when they would arrive. Often, they were only given a one-week "look ahead" that a shipment was on its way. This made it difficult to plan, even in jurisdictions that already had hospitals or health centers with the refrigeration and technology set up to administer vaccines. It was doubly difficult for rural areas without hospital facilities because they were served by mobile units and local recreational centers that required additional advance planning. It was very challenging to have some number of vaccine doses arrive at a rural medical facility without having the means to distribute them to a far-flung population.

By early January, it was clear that vaccine distribution at the state level had become a free-for-all. For example, New Jersey had set up a vaccine registration system using a third-party vendor. The original idea was that residents should sign up for it, and they would then be notified when they were eligible for the vaccine. But the registration system was quickly overwhelmed by thousands of would-be registrants. People seeking the vaccine then resorted to calling the number listed on the website, which in turn was overwhelmed by callers and long wait times. Moreover, the online system had been set up to weed out those who might have medical complications and provide them with instructions to contact their physicians for further guidance. But local physicians had no information to offer their patients. As a result, many people eligible for early vaccination were blocked by the registration system. Public health officials in New Jersey responded to this by allocating vaccines to the counties, some of which created their own megasites for vaccine distribution. Each distribution site created its own registration system. By January 2021, there were a bewildering variety of registration processes, each of which took time to fill out and each of which had to be checked individually by those seeking the vaccines.

The online registration systems were particularly hard on the most vulnerable populations, those over 75 years of age. Many seniors had neither the technology nor the computer skills to go online on multiple registration systems to seek for available vaccine distribution centers. As one editorial put it, "As of Saturday, Jan. 23, [2021,] the only place a Bergen County senior who was notified by the state to make that appointment could get a shot on that site was in Gloucester County. . . . An Essex County resident who got the 'schedule-now' email from the state was told that same day that there were no vaccine appointments available to him anywhere in New Jersey. The huge Kearny vaccination site would only serve those who live or work in Hudson County so if you're retired and live in North Arlington, good luck. The Middlesex County site didn't discriminate by county, but had no appointments available. Hackensack Meridian Health's website repeatedly told seniors to try again tomorrow. The Meadowlands site, also run by Hackensack Meridian, was completely booked as soon as it opened" (DiTommaso, 2021).

By early 2021 it also had become clear that racial disparities in vaccine administration were following the existing racial disparities in America's health care system overall, with white patients receiving the vaccines at a rate far exceeding that of African American patients. By March 2021, 13 percent of the white population in the United States had received at least one dose of a COVID-19 vaccine, in contrast to only 7 percent of the African American population. By April 2021, 33 percent of the white population had received at least one dose, in contrast to only 20 percent of the African American population.

Many cities with large populations of people of color made extra efforts to reach underserved populations, but that effort faced its own challenges.

In Philadelphia, racial disparities were especially sharp: in early February, 55 percent of those who had received the vaccination were white, even though they made up only 40 percent of the city's population. The city put out a call for companies that would prioritize testing and vaccination of underserved neighborhoods. City officials awarded a contract to a group called Philly Fighting COVID, led by a 22-year-old college graduate with no medical training and staffed by undergraduates even more inexperienced. This effort erupted into scandal when the company proved to be more interested in entrepreneurship than vaccinating at-risk patients.

In the wake of the scandal, a community-based group, the Black Doctors COVID-19 Consortium, received permission to hold the city's first walk-in vaccination clinic. In just over 24 hours, from February 24 through February 25, the consortium's doctors and staff vaccinated over 4,000 patients, approximately 80 percent of whom were people of color from some of the city's most vulnerable neighborhoods. Despite freezing rain and long lines, the event was successful, not only in the numbers vaccinated but also in showing that walk-in clinics could make a difference to many patients and communities.

In February 2021, President Joe Biden's newly installed administration had appointed new leadership in key federal agencies to expand and coordinate infrastructure for vaccine distribution. Perhaps the single most important measure taken was empowering the Federal Emergency Management Administration to work closely with nonfederal jurisdictions to set up and coordinate vaccination centers, and to deploy over 6,000 supporting personnel from agencies such as the Army and Navy Medical Corps and the National Guard. State, local, and regional jurisdictions were given reliable estimates of vaccines shipments three weeks in advance, so they could plan for the most effective distribution.

Among the most significant efforts was a new partnership between the Centers for Disease Control and Prevention and major retail pharmacy chains, including CVS, Rite Aid, Walmart, Walgreens, and Sam's Club. By mid-February, large shipments of the vaccines were put in the hands of people who routinely administered flu shots and other types of vaccinations. Vaccines were thus made accessible to millions of people in rural and urban areas alike. As CVS executives noted, 80 percent of Americans live within 10 miles of a CVS. Walmart noted that 70 percent of Americans live with five miles of a Walmart. Walmart made special efforts to reach underserved communities, partnering with community groups, setting up vaccination clinics in senior centers, and creating a fleet of mobile clinics to reach patients in the most remote areas. Jurisdictions continued to look for ways to deliver vaccines to more isolated groups, such as home-bound seniors or people with disabilities.

On April 19, 2021, all adults 16 and over were declared eligible for the vaccine. The GAO expressed confidence that federal agencies, working with state, Tribal, territorial, and local jurisdictions, could carry out the remainder of the distribution according to best practices of public health administration. That confidence was justified over the rest of the year, as COVID-19 vaccines became readily available in all U.S. health care jurisdictions.

FURTHER READING

DiTommaso, Lois. 2021. "New Jersey's Vaccine Rollout for Seniors a Massive Failure | Opinion." *NJ.com*. https://www.nj.com/opinion/2021/01/new-jerseys-vaccine-rollout-for-seniors-a-massive-failure-opinion.html.

Ndugga, Nambi, Olivia Pham, Latoya Hill, Samantha Artiga, Raisa Alam, and Noah Parker. 2021. "Latest Data on COVID-19 Vaccinations Race/Ethnicity." *KFF*. https://www.kff.org/coronavirus-covid-19/issue-brief/latest-data-on-covid-19-vaccinations-race-ethnicity.

Pegus, Cheryl. 2021. "Walmart Inc Now Offering Vaccines in 48 States, Puerto Rico, and Washington, DC." *Walmart.com*. https://corporate.walmart.com/newsroom/2021/04/02/walmart-inc-now-offering-covid-19-vaccines-in-48-states-puerto-rico-and-washington-d-c.

Reyes, Juliana Feliciano, Ellie Silverman, Ellie Rushing, and Oona Goodin-Smith. 2021. "How Philly Fighting Covid's Vaccine Effort Collapsed on a National Stage." *Philadelphia Inquirer*. https://www.inquirer.com/health/coronavirus/philly-fighting-covid-vaccine-signup-andrei-doroshin-20210131.html.

Rushing, Ellie, Oona Goodin-Smith, and Anna Orso. 2021. "Philly Black Doctors Clinic Outpaced the City in Vaccinating Black Residents, but Group Says There's 'Room for Improvement.'" *Philadelphia Inquirer*. https://www.inquirer.com/health/coronavirus/philadelphia-coronavirus-vaccine-black-doctors-covid-consortium-20210225.html.

US Government Accountability Office. 2020. "COVID-19. Federal Efforts Could Be Strengthened by Timely and Concerted Actions." GAO-20-701. https://www.gao.gov/products/gao-20-701.

US Government Accountability Office. 2021. "COVID-19. Efforts to Increase Vaccine Availability and Perspectives on Initial Implementation." GAO-21-443. https://www.gao.gov/products/gao-21-443.

Q13. DID VACCINE HESITANCY INTERFERE WITH COVID-19 VACCINE DISTRIBUTION IN THE UNITED STATES?

Answer: That depends. Vaccine hesitancy, defined by the World Health Organization (WHO) as "delay in acceptance or refusal of vaccines despite availability of vaccination services," was certainly a factor in keeping vaccination acceptance rates in some regions below the percentage recommended by public health officials in order to establish herd immunity. However, vaccine hesitancy proved to be less of a factor than had been predicted at the start of the pandemic. From December 2020 through December 2021, a much higher percentage of the population was vaccinated against COVID-19 than receives the flu vaccine during a typical year.

Sadly, however, those who chose not to be vaccinated were at much greater risk for dangerous symptoms and hospitalization when the Delta and Omicron variants of COVID-19 spread from the summer of 2021 through the winter of 2022.

Vaccine hesitancy did not start with the COVID-19 vaccines, however. The definition above came from the 2014 report of the WHO working group on vaccination hesitancy, published after three years of research and deliberation. The group noted that both the causes and consequences of vaccine hesitancy were complicated, and that they varied across time and geographical location. Moreover, hesitancy exists on a continuum between outright acceptance—people who want all available vaccines—and outright refusal—people who refuse all vaccines. Most people are hesitant about some vaccines and accepting of others. They may, for example, be willing to get a rabies shot if they work with animals but refuse a routine flu shot as unnecessary.

Vaccine hesitancy only comes into play when the vaccine in question is readily available to everyone who wants them. It does not refer to situations where people cannot get vaccinated because of what the report called system failures: "lack of vaccine, stock-outs, lack of vaccine offer, infeasible travel/ distances to reach immunization clinics, missing vaccine program communication, or curtailment of vaccine services in the presence of conflict, natural disaster or similar situations" (WHO, 2014). In all those cases, it's not concerns about the vaccine itself, but rather the hardships involved in getting them, that is the reason for the refusal.

The decision to be vaccinated or not is often perceived by vaccine-hesitant people as their own individual choice. In most countries, that choice is reinforced by laws allowing patients to refuse as well as accept health care. However, under COVID-19 conditions, vaccine hesitancy became part of larger public and private discussions about the best way to end the pandemic and return to normal life.

The Facts: During the fall of 2020, as the COVID-19 vaccines were in development, concerns about vaccine hesitancy and its potential impact on a vaccine rollout became part of public discourse. According to CDC analysis, 85 percent of the United States population would have to either contract and recover from COVID-19 or receive the vaccine in order for the country to achieve herd immunity, so that the virus would no longer be able to spread to vulnerable people. However, publicly available data indicated that only approximately 45 percent of Americans received a flu vaccine in any given year. The numbers varied by state, ranging from 38 percent to 55 percent. They varied by race, age, and income as well, and there were also disparities between rural areas on the one hand, and urban and suburban areas on the other.

If COVID-19 vaccinations followed those patterns, it would be impossible to achieve herd immunity. The virus would become endemic, with frequent flare-ups in coming years—similar to flu outbreaks but with much higher morbidity and mortality. Large numbers of unvaccinated people also made it much more likely that the COVID-19 virus would develop variants. Existing and new variants would spread to vulnerable patients and become endemic in their turn.

COVID-19 vaccines were distributed in phases set by the CDC in conjunction with other public health officials. Each phase indicated the groups that would be eligible. Phase 1a, initiated as of December 3, 2020, included health care personnel and residents of long-term care facilities. Health care personnel were eligible in this first phase because they were the most vulnerable in treating COVID-19 patients. It included not only doctors and nurses, but also support staff in hospitals and medical centers who provided food and janitorial services for patients. Residents of long-term care facilities had been shown to be dangerously vulnerable to infection; the new vaccine would save not only their lives but also those of others who came into contact with them. It would also pave the way for reopening the facilities for visitors, thus ending the tragic isolation of residents from families.

Phases 1b and 1c were announced on December 22, 2020. Phase 1b included frontline essential workers, including firefighters, police officers, U.S. Postal Service workers, grocery store workers, and transit workers. Phase 1c included people aged 65–74 years of age, as well as people aged 16–64 with health conditions that made them more vulnerable to severe cases of COVID-19. By March 2021, as more doses of vaccine became available, many jurisdictions added more categories, such as teachers and support staff in educational settings. By April 16, when vaccine eligibility was opened to anyone over age 16, analysts estimated that the United States was on track to provide the vaccines to everyone who wanted them by the end of May.

Yet even though health care personnel were among the first groups eligible for the vaccine, by March 2020, only a little over 50 percent had been vaccinated. Approximately 30 percent were either hesitant about getting the vaccine or did not want it at all (Dror, 2020). Moreover, there were clear disparities in vaccination attitudes depending on education and income. Over 70 percent of health care personnel with graduate degrees—including doctors, physician assistants, and senior staff—were eager to get the vaccine, as were over 60 percent of those with bachelor's degrees. In contrast, only approximately 40 percent of those with associate's degree's or less, including junior nursing staff, janitorial, and food-service workers, intended to be vaccinated. The same kind of leveling-off process could be seen when health care personnel were grouped by income. Almost 70 percent of those earning more than $90,000 were vaccinated or intended to be. In contrast, only about half of those in the $40,000–$90,000 range, and only about 30 percent of those earning under $40,000, wanted the vaccines (Dror, 2020).

The kind of health care facility at which workers were employed made a difference as well. Vaccination rates were highest in facilities that offered their employees the vaccine. In hospitals, 66 percent of staff received the vaccine, in contrast to just around 50 percent of those who worked in long-term care facilities, 39 percent of those who were self-employed, and 26 percent of those who worked in private homes (Wan, 2021).

The reasons given by the first batch of health care workers for their hesitancy about getting vaccinated against COVID-19 were echoed again and again in subsequent surveys. They included fears that the vaccine had been developed too quickly and without enough time for safety trials. They were concerned about side effects. Many said that they were waiting to see how the vaccines affected others, particularly others "like them"—that is, not the rich and famous, but rather people of their own race, ethnicity, occupation, and income level.

By March 2021, the vaccines became more widely available in more convenient settings. This environment provided the precondition for true vaccine hesitancy according to the WHO definition: "delay or refusal" to get vaccinated despite "availability of vaccination services." As a number of surveys found, although vaccine hesitancy was not be as high as originally feared, it was still a significant public health issue. According to Kaiser Family Foundation polls, 66 percent of those surveyed either had gotten the vaccine or intended to, up from 61 percent a month earlier; the number of "undecideds" had dropped from 18 percent to 14 percent, and even the number of those who were unwilling to be vaccinated had dropped, from 21 percent to 20 percent. The shift was particularly striking among certain categories of respondents. Early surveys had noted a marked disparity between Democrats and Republicans, with only 25 percent of Democrats expressing hesitancy about the vaccine in mid-March, while 47 percent of Republicans did so. By mid-April, the hesitancy among Democrats had shifted downward to 21 percent, while the hesitancy among Republicans had dropped to 41 percent. While still significantly higher than among Democrats, the GOP numbers were roughly comparable to the numbers among Independents, whose hesitancy rate had fallen from 42 percent to 38 percent (Hamel, 2021a).

A key factor affecting vaccine hesitancy was age. Eighty-five percent of those aged 65 and older either had the vaccine or planned to get it, with only 6 percent expressing uncertainty and 9 percent unwilling to be vaccinated. In obvious contrast, 54 percent of those in the 18–34 age group had been or planned to be vaccinated, with 21 percent uncertain and 27 percent unwilling. For the younger age group, the most common reason given was that they did not believe they were at high risk for COVID-19. At every age group, the higher the income, the greater the willingness to be vaccinated. Higher educational levels also equated to greater willingness to be vaccinated (Hamel, 2021b).

There were also disparities among people in different occupational groups. By April 2021, the occupational group with the highest percentage of people either already or intending to be vaccinated—80 percent—were educators and child care workers. This is particularly impressive as in many states, people in those occupations only became eligible at the beginning of March. Those who worked in technology or financial services also reported high levels of interest in vaccination, with 79 percent and 74 percent vaccine acceptance. By November 2021, 76 percent of health care workers were either vaccinated or intending to be. Those employed in food and beverage services, construction, and agriculture had the lowest rate of vaccine acceptance—71 percent, 65 percent, and 56 percent, respectively ("Vaccine Sentiment Dashboard," 2021).

It seems likely that for the occupational groups with lowest rates of vaccine acceptance, concerns about side effects were combined with a lack of access to the vaccines during their ordinary working day. Employees in those groups often had to leave their workplace to travel to vaccine distribution centers, and they might have to take additional time off to deal with side effects. In contrast, those employed in technology or financial services were often located closer to vaccine distribution centers. They also were more likely to have benefits such as paid sick leave they could draw on to get the vaccine and recover from any side effects.

Public health agencies and private companies worked together to address vaccine hesitancy by promoting positive messaging. The Ad Council, an organization with a long history of harnessing the power of advertising for social causes, created the COVID-19 Vaccine Education Initiative to encourage vaccination. Many companies offered incentives, such as increased vacation days or cash bonuses, to encourage their employees to "get vaxxed." Local public health agencies reached out to religious leaders within their communities and arranged for faith-based community centers to become vaccination sites. Media celebrities and political leaders with large public followings proclaimed their vaccination status and urged their fans and supporters to get the COVID-19 vaccine. In New York, public health officials arranged for pop-up vaccination centers in train and subway stations, with free commuter tickets as giveaways; tourists were invited to be vaccinated for free in Times Square. Ohio was the first state to offer lottery tickets for a jackpot of $1 million as an incentive for vaccination; when the number of vaccinations shot up, other states followed suit.

Between March and November 2021, the overall rate of COVID-19 vaccine hesitancy in the United States dropped from 39 percent to 27 percent of the adult population ("Vaccine Sentiment Dashboard," 2021). The close study of vaccine hesitancy during the COVID-19 pandemic reinforces previous research findings: that more people are willing to be vaccinated when there is a clear and present health crisis; when there is loud, frequent, and consistent positive messaging about vaccination; and when there is clear evidence that vaccination is effective in protecting them and their families. It reinforces other findings as well, for example, that people are more motivated by the desire to protect their health and return to normal life than by public service messages about preventing transmission to other people. Finally, it shows how hard it is to separate ease of access from willingness to be vaccinated: overall, those groups who had easier, more convenient access to vaccines with supportive environments at work and at home were more likely to decide in favor of being vaccinated.

FURTHER READING

Ad Council. 2021. "Covid-19 Vaccine Education Initiative." https://www.adcouncil.org/covid-vaccine.

Dror, Amiel A., Netanel Eisenbach, Shahar Taiber, Nicole G. Morozov, Matti Mizrachi, Asaf Zigron, Samer Srouji, and Eyal Sela. 2020. "Vaccine Hesitancy: The Next Challenge in the Fight against COVID-19."

European Journal of Epidemiology 35: 775–79. https://doi.org/10.1007/s10654-020-00671-y.

Hamel, Liz, Grace Sparks, and Mollyann Brodie. 2021a. "Vaccine Confidence, Intentions and Trends." *KFF.org.* https://www.kff.org/coronavirus-covid-19/poll-finding/kff-covid-19-vaccine-monitor-february-2021/.

Hamel, Liz, Lunna Lopez, Grace Sparks, Mellisha Stokes, and Mollyann Brodie. 2021b. "KFF Covid Vaccine Monitor: April 2021." *KFF.org.* https://www.kff.org/coronavirus-covid-19/poll-finding/kff-covid-19-vaccine-monitor-april-2021/.

Hoffman, Jan. 2021. "Clergy Preach Faith in the Covid Vaccine to Doubters." *New York Times.* https://www.nytimes.com/2021/03/14/health/clergy-covid-vaccine.html.

Rosenbaum, Lisa. 2021. "Escaping Catch-22—Overcoming Covid Vaccine Hesitancy." *New England Journal of Medicine* 384: 1367–71. https://www.nejm.org/doi/full/10.1056/NEJMms2101220.

"Vaccine Sentiment Dashboard." 2021. *Morning Consult.* https://morningconsult.com/covid19-vaccine-dashboard.

Wan, William, Frances Stead Sellers, Naema Ahmed, and Emily Guskin. 2021. "More Than 4 in 10 Health-Care Workers Have Not Been Vaccinated, Post-KFF Poll Finds." *Washington Post.* https://www.washingtonpost.com/health/2021/03/19/health-workers-covid-vaccine.

World Health Organization (WHO). 2014. "Report of the SAGE Working Group on Vaccine Hesitancy." https://www.who.int/immunization/sage/meetings/2014/october/1_Report_WORKING_GROUP_vaccine_hesitancy_final.pdf.

Q14. DID FRAUD AND DISINFORMATION HAVE AN IMPACT ON COVID-19 VACCINE DISTRIBUTION?

Answer: Yes. Unfortunately, the COVID-19 pandemic, like many crises, provided opportunities for bad actors to try to take advantage of people for their own personal gain. Their activities included exploiting social media practices to drive traffic to their websites, outright fraud such as fake vaccination cards, and even attempts to sell fraudulent vaccines.

Fortunately, cybersecurity experts and federal and local law enforcement issues were able to prevent the worst of the scams. Schemes for selling fraudulent vaccines were shut down well before the products reached any potential patients, and although some fake vaccination cards may have been sold, they do not seem to have had any impact on public health.

Disinformation was more of a challenge. According to the useful definition developed by the Pacific Science Center, "Misinformation is incorrect information shared by mistake. Disinformation is incorrect information shared deliberately" (Pacific Science Center, 2020). The World Health Organization (WHO) declared the volume of mis- and disinformation an "infodemic," and public health and cybersecurity organizations worldwide worked on strategies to counteract it. This included careful monitoring of social media outlets, education initiatives for consumers, and even the development of online games to teach children—and their parents—to recognize COVID-19 disinformation.

The Facts: As the COVID-19 vaccines were in development in the fall of 2020, the United States Department of Homeland Security worked together with Interpol and other international security agencies to protect the public against anticipated vaccine fraud and scams. The vaccines were expected to be a valuable commodity worldwide, making them perfect targets for criminal activity, including the production and sale of counterfeit vaccine materials and an array of internet scams designed to steal money or personal information.

As Mike Alfonso of Homeland Security Investigations explained, his agency has broad responsibility for protecting the United States against many different kinds of criminal activity. At the beginning of the COVID-19 pandemic, they realized that the rapid development of all types of new products, from personal protective equipment (PPE) to therapeutics to vaccines, could all too easily turn out to be a fraudster's dream and a consumer's nightmare. The agency therefore launched Operation Stolen Promise, consisting of investigators, cyber security experts, and financial agents, to combat illegal activity emerging from the pandemic. As the vaccines were under development, they worked closely with pharmaceutical companies to ensure that they fully understood the products they needed to protect. They spoke to research scientists, manufacturers, and even marketing and design professionals to ensure they knew exactly what the vaccine should look like, how it should be packaged, and how to distinguish between genuine company trademarks and logos and their counterfeits. They also carefully examined all aspects of the supply chain, including shipping and storage aspects, to make sure that they were protected from break-ins or hijacking.

Alfonso and his international colleagues were extremely successful in protecting the genuine vaccines: there were no reported cases of theft of any of the millions of doses shipped worldwide. Within the United States, they were also successful in preventing the importation or distribution of counterfeit vaccines. Overseas, Interpol identified two crime rings involved in distributing fake vaccines. One, in South Africa, resulted in the seizure of 2,400 doses of counterfeit vaccine and the arrest of four suspects. Another Interpol investigation in China ended in the seizure of 3,000 fake vaccine doses and the arrest of around 80 suspects. To alert people to potential fraud, Interpol issued a set of public service graphics warning consumers against vaccine scams with the tagline "Be vigilant. Be skeptical. Be safe."

Most criminals stayed away from creating and selling counterfeit vaccines because that type of fraud required financial outlays for realistic-looking bottles and fluid that could be passed off as genuine vaccine. Instead, most criminals preferred the tried-and-true strategies of internet fraud. As Alfonso noted, the most prevalent form of fraud in the early days of the vaccines were fake websites offering to sell vaccines directly to consumers. These websites falsely claimed that the vaccines they were selling came directly from pharmaceutical companies, like Moderna and Pfizer. Homeland Security investigators worked to shut them down as quickly as possible, warning the public that no legitimate vaccines were ever for sale online.

Once the vaccines were available, scammers switched to a new type of fraud. They emailed surveys to patients, asking them for information on their vaccination experience. These surveys were made to look as if they came from reputable vaccine manufacturers. Sometimes these scams offered an iPad or other consumer product as a prize for filling out the survey, but with the catch that the email recipient had to supply credit card information to have the product shipped. Again, law enforcement officials warned, no legitimate company would ever send a survey that requested personal information. All legitimate research surveys have protocols in place to keep personal information private.

As vaccinations became common, scammers developed still another way to defraud the public—selling fake vaccination cards. Public health officials had not originally given much thought to designing or protecting vaccination cards, as their only legitimate purpose was to serve as a reminder of the type of vaccine and date for the second dose of the Pfizer and Moderna vaccines. They were created out of stiff paper with handwritten information, just like standard appointment cards that patients often receive from their doctors. Hundreds of accounts on shopping sites like Shopify and eBay attempted to sell blank vaccination cards. One seller was marketing a set of four blank vaccination cards for $80. Though all such accounts were shut down as soon as the sites were made aware of them, the same seller might pop-up with a new account elsewhere.

In March 2021, the FBI issued a special public service announcement, warning that making and buying fake COVID-19 vaccination record cards was a danger to the public and a violation of the law. Legitimate vaccination record cards were issued by the Centers for Disease Control and Prevention, and falsifying them could carry the same penalty as falsifying other kinds of government documents. "If you did not receive the vaccine," the FBI warned, **"do not make your own vaccine cards, and do not fill-in blank vaccination record cards with false information"** (FBI, 2021).

Disinformation posed a challenge of a different kind. Law enforcement officials cannot do very much about people who deliberately circulate wrong or misleading information, unless they are making incorrect claims directly about a product they are trying to sell. But even if they are posting disinformation online to entice consumers to click through to a shopping website, that may fall outside the purview of law enforcement. It is an extension of the marketing strategy known as clickbait, in which online marketers or influencers use attention-grabbing links to entice viewers to their websites. It has been shown to work particularly well with news items that are sensational and provoke strong negative emotions, like fear and anxiety. A phrase like "Dangerous New Finding," accompanied by a frightening image, will attract more clicks than "Celebrating my COVID shot" with smiley faces.

The combination of the pandemic with the widespread use of social media created ripe conditions for an infodemic, defined by WHO as "an overabundance of information, both online and offline. It includes deliberate attempts to disseminate wrong information to undermine the public health response and advance alternative agendas of groups or individuals."

Due to the power of social media to influence public opinion, these deliberate attempts could do a great deal of harm. "Misinformation costs lives," WHO warned. "Without the appropriate trust and correct information, diagnostic tests go unused, immunization campaigns (or campaigns to promote effective vaccines) will not meet their targets, and the virus will continue to thrive" (WHO, September 2020). Public health officials were especially concerned that disinformation campaigns would increase vaccine hesitancy and thus increase the risk that COVID-19 variants could become endemic in the population, leading to higher-than-necessary mortality and morbidity for years to come.

Disinformation campaigns against COVID-19 vaccines tapped into well-known features of online behavior. One is fearmongering. Posts that create or tap into fears are known to get more clicks than those that express happiness or contentment. Those that express outrage have also been shown to get more clicks than those that express nuance or thoughtful concern. Other strategies include highlighting authorities or trusted public figures who support the point of view presented in the post—or inventing experts to support their positions if none exist.

Controversy is another mechanism for generating web traffic, and disinformation providers may link to already-controversial posts to piggyback onto existing links. They may demonize prominent researchers and celebrities and attack them online, again with the strategy of generating traffic. They may take information from legitimate websites and twist it to serve their own purposes. And they may do all of this while using personas that make them seem like actual people—concerned moms, for instance—when in fact they are really a particularly unscrupulous set of internet marketers. Indeed, studies have shown that many disinformation sites contain posts generated by bots, self-running software designed to create the illusion of an actual internet community.

Reports on COVID-19 disinformation from June through August 2020, before the vaccines were available, showed that it flourished in areas where there were "data deficits," that is, a lack of reliable information from trusted sources. This was a period when concerns about the newness of the vaccines and their safety and accuracy were particularly strong. Many disinformation sites posed as legitimate sources of information in order to generate traffic. They often featured "zombie" content, false information about earlier vaccines that had been circulating in digital and legacy formats—in some cases for decades. And they plagiarized and distorted legitimate, responsible news sources presenting nuanced information, in order to heighten fears that the vaccines would not be properly tested or equitably distributed.

WHO and other public health agencies worked together with responsible journalists and advertisers to educate the public on how to protect themselves against disinformation. They developed seven steps for consumers: (1) Assess the source, (2) go beyond headlines, (3) identify the author, (4) check the date, (5) examine the supporting evidence, (6) check your biases, and (7) turn to fact-checkers. Short games such as Go Viral were developed to help educate young people on how disinformation posts work.

The most effective strategy for dealing with COVID-19 disinformation, however, was the decision by top social media platforms to flag it or shut it down. Google, Facebook, Twitter, and YouTube worked to flag COVID-19 disinformation when posted by legitimate users, and they also adopted policies to shut down sites run by known bad actors or populated by bots. YouTube alone removed 30,000 misleading COVID-19 vaccine videos in the first five months of the vaccine distribution. Studies of online behavior found that flagging posts with warnings of misleading COVID-19 content had a significant impact on viewers' perceptions, and it was thus an effective technique in fighting disinformation.

FURTHER READING

Cerullo, Megan. 2021. "Scammers Are Selling Fake COVID-19 Vaccination Cards Online." *CBS News*. https://www.cbsnews.com/news/covid-vaccination-cards-fake-scammers-fraud.

Federal Bureau of Investigation (FBI) Public Service Announcement. 2021. "If You Make or Buy a Fake COVID-19 Vaccination Record Card, You Endanger Yourself and Those around You, and You Are Breaking the Law." Alert Number I-033021-PSA, March 30, 2021. https://www.ic3.gov/Media/Y2021/PSA210330.

Go Viral! 2020. https://www.goviralgame.com/en.

Interpol. 2021. "Online Vaccine Scams: INTERPOL and Homeland Security Investigations Issue Public Warning." https://www.interpol.int/en/News-and-Events/News/2021/Online-vaccine-scams-INTERPOL-and-Homeland-Security-Investigations-issue-public-warning.

Marshall, Serena, and Lara Salah. 2021. "Buyer Beware: Fighting COVID Vaccine Fraud." *Medpage Today*. https://www.medpagetoday.com/podcasts/trackthevax/91862.

Pacific Science Center. 2020. "Facts in the Time of Covid." https://view.genial.ly/5eea3a0c15e1e60d88c5c4d0/interactive-content-facts-in-the-time-of-covid-19.

Smith, Rory, Seb Cubbon, and Claire Wardle. 2021. "Under the Surface: Covid-19 Vaccine Narratives, Misinformation and Data Deficits on Social Media." *First Draft*. https://firstdraftnews.org/long-form-article/under-the-surface-covid-19-vaccine-narratives-misinformation-and-data-deficits-on-social-media/.

Steele, Jim. 2021. "Flagging Coronavirus Misinformation Tweets Changes User Behaviors, New Research Shows." *University of Alabama in Huntsville News*. https://www.uah.edu/news/news/flagging-coronavirus-misinformation-tweets-changes-user-behaviors-new-research-shows.

World Health Organization (WHO). n.d. "Let's flatten the infodemic curve." Accessed May 1, 2021. https://www.who.int/news-room/spotlight/let-s-flatten-the-infodemic-curve.

World Health Organization (WHO). 2020. "Managing the COVID-19 Infodemic: Promoting Healthy Behaviours and Mitigating the Harm from Misinformation and Disinformation." https://www.who.int/news/item/23-09-2020-managing-the-covid-19-infodemic-promoting-healthy-behaviours-and-mitigating-the-harm-from-misinformation-and-disinformation.

Q15. DID THE SPREAD OF VARIANT STRAINS HAVE AN IMPACT ON THE COVID-19 PANDEMIC?

Answer: Yes. Coronaviruses, like other viruses, can quickly develop mutations. Many of these mutations are not viable—that is, the virus strains that develop them are unable to reproduce. Those that are viable because they can reproduce are known as variants. These variants have the same basic molecular structure, but they differ in certain parts of their genetic code, and these differences may affect the way they interact with their hosts. Modern techniques in computational biology—computers applied to biological research—have made it possible to identify and sequence viruses in real time during outbreaks and to track variants as they develop.

Within six months of the start of the COVID-19 outbreak, careful research and surveillance showed that variants of the original SARS-CoV-2 strain were spreading. They quickly became a focal point for investigation, because no one knew the impact these variants could have. Would the variants be more or less infectious than the original strain? Would patients develop more or less severe symptoms, and be at greater or lesser risk of serious illness or death? And would existing vaccines, and those already under development, protect patients against the new variants?

The four variants that garnered most attention were initially named after the locations in which they were first identified, but they were later given location-neutral names according to the Greek alphabet. Throughout 2021, the Delta variant had the greatest impact. Studies showed that it led to more severe symptoms than the original strain, and it was twice as infectious. By the spring of 2021, the Delta variant was increasingly responsible for new cases worldwide. By July 2021, it was the dominant strain in the United States, and it was responsible for the spike in new cases, hospitalizations, and deaths throughout the summer. Though the U.S. infection rate had slowed to a seven-day moving average of 12,000 in June, it was up to 60,000 by the end of July.

The greatest risk from the Delta variant was to unvaccinated people. Spikes in new COVID-19 cases throughout the world were correlated with countries and regions where vaccination rates were low. Unvaccinated people died of the Delta variant at a rate 10 times that of vaccinated people. Unvaccinated people were 11 times more likely to be hospitalized and 5 times more likely to be infected (Dyer, 2021).

Still, the rapid spread of the Delta variant also affected those who were vaccinated, leading to "breakthrough infections." That is the term used for patients who tested positive for COVID-19 after being fully vaccinated. By the end of 2021, the Food and Drug Administration authorized booster shots for the Pfizer/BioNTech, Moderna, and Johnson & Johnson vaccines as a response to the Delta variant.

The Delta variant had a direct impact on vaccinations in the United States as well. From June 2021 through August 2021, there was an uptick in the number of people seeking vaccinations. Surveys showed that fears of the Delta variant, the increase in hospitalizations, and personal connections to those who had become ill or died were the most frequent reasons given by people who decided to be vaccinated over the summer.

In November 2021, public health authorities in South Africa reported a new variant of concern, B.1.1.529, which was given the name Omicron. By January 6, it had been reported in 149 countries. In the United States, it became the leading variant, responsible for an estimated 95% of new cases. Omicron was much more transmissable than the Delta variant and led to an increase in breakthrough infections (Accorsi, 2022).

While even fully vaccinated people were more susceptible to the Omicron than the Delta variant, CDC studies found that the vaccines were highly effective in preventing dangerous diseases. Unvaccinated people were 12 times as likely to test positive for Omicron than those who were vaccinated, and 83 times more likely to be hospitalized. Previously-vaccinated patients who tested positive for Omicron were also less likely to spread the disease to others (Danza, 2022).

The Facts: Viruses mutate all the time, and health officials estimate that there are thousands of variants of the SARS-CoV-2 circulating around the globe. Most are inconsequential and have no noticeable difference on patients: the variant strains cannot be distinguished from the original strain except through DNA sequencing. Some, though, do seem to behave differently when interacting with the human population. These are the ones that are most important to monitor. They may be less responsive to COVID-19 testing, making them harder to screen for. They may be less likely to be neutralized by antibodies created by previous infection or through vaccination. Treatments known to work against the original strain may be less effective. If the immune system and known treatments are less able to defend the body against the variants, they may spread more rapidly or to more vulnerable populations.

The more a virus spreads, the more opportunities it has to develop viable mutations that can become variants. Evolutionary pressures affect the nature of the mutations: a slight change in the complex genetic code that can help a virus spread to more people, or resist antibodies, will help a virus strain with that genetic change to survive and become a stable variant.

The Centers for Disease Control and Prevention (CDC) developed a classification scheme that identified variants by their anticipated impact on public health. The first category, variants of interest, were those whose genetic characteristics had been found to affect the way the variants respond to prevention—including social distancing as well as vaccination—and treatment. They might create clusters of the disease in specific populations, but appeared to be limited in how far they spread. The second category, variants of concern, are more severe in their impact: they differ more from the known behaviors of the original strain, and they can cause more severe disease. The third category, variants of high importance, differ enough from the existing strain that testing, prevention, and treatment measures put into place no longer work against it. Fortunately, no variants of high importance were identified for the SARS-CoV-2 virus.

The variants of concern all have small mutations in the spike protein that make them more effective in infecting humans. The Alpha (scientific designation: B.1.1.7) is more infectious than the original strain, and it subsequently spread to 50 countries. The Beta (B.1.351) and Gamma (P.1) variants have mutations that help the virus evade antibodies. They spread to 20 and 10 countries, respectively. The Delta and Omicron variants (B.1.617.2 and B.1.1.529) were the most infectious, and they spread worldwide. All of these are common adaptations among viruses. The mutations don't change the nature of the virus—for example, a coronavirus doesn't suddenly change from being a respiratory disease to causing cancer. Instead, the mutations help the virus become more effective at attacking patients' cells, resisting the immune system, and spreading from person to person.

The vaccines first distributed in the winter of 2020–21 had been developed to work against the original strain of SRS-CoV-2, and so scientists paid close attention to how effective they were against variants. By May 2021, preliminary studies showed that the new vaccines were still highly effective against the Alpha, Beta, and Gamma variants. They were slightly less effective against the Delta variant, and that finding was confirmed by September 2021.

While this might seem to be bad news—no one wants the COVID-19 virus to win its battle against humans by mutating—it is not as bad as it may seem at first. In studying the impact of the vaccines against the variants, scientists looked at two types of efficacy: how effective vaccination was at preventing people from getting sick at all, and how effective it was at preventing people from experiencing severe symptoms. As with many kinds of illnesses, patients who contracted COVID-19 experienced a range of symptoms, with some people having mild or no effects from the disease, and other suffering from very severe effects that led to hospitalization and even death. While the first set of vaccines did not completely protect patients from breakthrough infections, they were still highly effective in preventing the most serious symptoms as well as in preventing the most serious outcomes: hospitalization and death.

Countries with the highest vaccination rates suffered less from the spread of the Delta variant. In December 2020, the Israeli Ministry of Health launched a far-reaching campaign to vaccinate the entire adult population of the country with the Pfizer-BioNTech vaccine. Israel had in place a very efficient system for data collection of new cases of COVID-19, of the virus variant that produced them, and of the vaccination efforts. At the time, 95 percent of the new cases were caused by the Alpha variant. Data based on this campaign, collected from January 4, 2021, through April 3, 2021, confirmed that two doses of the Pfizer-BioNTech vaccine had efficacy rates in actual use that matched the efficacy rates in the clinical trials. The efficacy rates against COVID-19 infections where patients exhibited symptoms was especially high, at 96 percent across all age groups, even patients between 75 and 85 years of age. Cases where patients do not exhibit symptoms are harder to assess, because asymptomatic patients may not have been tested unless they were in an occupation that required routine testing, such as education, health care, or the military. Even with this qualification, the study showed the vaccines had an efficacy rate of over 90 percent against asymptomatic COVID-19 infections.

Where breakthrough infections did occur after vaccination, they came either in the period between the first and second shot, or within two weeks of the second shot. This, too, had been predicted by the clinical trials, because the data showed that the vaccines took until two weeks after the second dose to reach maximum effect. Those who were infected a week after the second dose were more likely to be infected with the Delta variant, suggesting that the virus mutation might have some small advantage over the original strain in its fight against the vaccine. But overall, the incidence of the Delta variant remained very low in Israel. The high efficacy of the Pfizer-BioNTech vaccines, coupled with the high efficacy of national vaccination efforts, limited the spread of variants that could cause dangerous symptoms.

To protect against variants, all vaccine manufacturers—Moderna, Johnson and Johnson, and Oxford/AstraZeneca including Pfizer-BioNTech—developed booster shots based on the specific characteristics of the variant strains of SARS-CoV-2. Booster shots are updated versions of a vaccine designed to "boost" the immunity of the patient, and they are common for childhood vaccines. Within the United States and elsewhere, public health officials developed expedited approval processes for the COVID booster shots, in case any of the variants of concern were to cause a new wave of infections. As the impact of the Delta variant became clear over the summer of 2021, boosters were made available to high-risk populations, including those 65 years of age and older; those in high-risk occupations like health care; those with frequent exposure to unvaccinated populations, such as teachers; and those aged 16 through 64 with underlying health conditions that made them most vulnerable to COVID-19. By December 2021, all U.S. adults were eligible for booster shots. News of the Omicron variant led to an uptick in vaccinations in January and February 2022.

Detecting and tracking variants depends on advanced gene-sequencing techniques, and that can create challenges for public health officials. Genetic sequencing has a high cost, as it requires specialized laboratories and trained specialist personnel. It also requires a lot of genetic material. Researchers have to have access to millions of samples of the pathogen, or the existing tests may not be able to detect variants. Gene sequencing has flourished during the COVID-19 pandemic.

As with any large-scale testing and aggregating of data, there are privacy concerns. Researchers who have access to data have to take every possible precaution to ensure that individuals whose pathogens are part of the study cannot be identified. The Israeli study, discussed above, stated explicitly, "Only aggregate data, with no personal identifiers, were used in this analysis" (Haas et al., 2021). CDC surveys have taken the same precautions. Cybersecurity experts have been part of the process to ensure that information about pathogens and their mutations does not fall into the hands of bad actors who might try to develop biological weapons.

FURTHER READING

Accorsi, Emma K., Amadea Britton, Katherine Fleming-Dutra, Zachary R. Smith, Nong Shang, Gordana Derado, Joseph Miller, Stephanie J. Schrag, and Jennifer R. Verani. 2022. "Association Between 3 Doses of mRNA COVID-19 Vaccine and Symptomatic Infection Caused by the SARS-CoV-2 Omicron and Delta Variants." *Journal of the American Medical Association* 327 (7): 639–51. https://dx.doi.org/10.1001/jama.2022.0470.

Centers for Disease Control and Prevention (CDC). 2021a. "Delta Variant: What We Know about the Science." Updated August 26, 2021. https://www.cdc.gov/coronavirus/2019-ncov/variants/delta-variant.html.

Centers for Disease Control and Prevention (CDC). 2021b. "What You Need to Know about the Variants." Updated September 20, 2021. https://www.cdc.gov/coronavirus/2019-ncov/variants/variant.html.

Danza, Phoebe, Tae Hee Koo, Meredith Haddix, Rebecca Fisher, Elizabeth Traub, Kelsey OYong, and Sharon Balter. 2022. "SARS-CoV-2 Infection and Hospitalization among Adults Aged ≥18 Years, by Vaccination Status, Before and During SARS-CoV-2 B.1.1.529 (Omicron) Variant Predominance—Los Angeles County, California, November 7, 2021– January 8, 2022." *Morbidity and Mortality Weekly Reports* 71 (5): 177–81. http://dx.doi.org/10.15585/mmwr.mm7105e1.

Dyer, Owen. 2021. "Covid-19: Unvaccinated Face 11 Times Risk of Death from Delta Variant, CDC Data Show." *British Medical Journal* 374 (September): n2282. https://doi.org/10.1136/bmj.n2282.

Haas, Eric, et al. 2021. "Impact and Effectiveness of mRNA BNT162b2 Vaccine Against SARS-CoV-2 Infections and COVID-19 Cases, Hospitalisations, and Deaths Following a Nationwide Vaccination Campaign in Israel: An Observational Study Using National Surveillance Data." *The Lancet.* https://www.thelancet.com/journals/lancet/article/PIIS0140-6736(21)00947-8/fulltext.

Irfan, Umair. 2021. "Will Covid-19 Vaccines Protect You against Variants? 9 Questions about Variants, Answered." *Vox.* https://www.vox.com/22385588/covid-19-vaccine-variant-mutation-n440k-india-moderna-pfizer-b1617.

Lesham, Eyal, and Annalies Wilder-Smith. 2021. "COVID-19 Vaccine Impact in Israel and a Way Out of the Pandemic." *The Lancet.* https://www.thelancet.com/journals/lancet/article/PIIS0140-6736(21)01018-7/fulltext.

"Surging Delta Variant Cases, Hospitalizations, and Deaths Are Biggest Drivers of Recent Uptick in U.S. COVID-19 Vaccination Rates." 2021. *Kaiser Family Foundation (KFF) Newsroom.* https://www.kff.org/coronavirus-covid-19/press-release/surging-delta-variant-cases-hospitalizations-and-deaths-are-biggest-drivers-of-recent-uptick-in-u-s-covid-19-vaccination-rates/.

U.S. Government Accountability Office. 2021. "Science & Tech Spotlight: Genomic Sequencing of Infectious Pathogens." GAO-21-426SP, March 30, 2021. https://www.gao.gov/assets/gao-21-426sp.pdf.

Q16. WERE SAFE COVID-19 VACCINES DEVELOPED FOR CHILDREN?

Answer: Yes. Shortly after Pfizer-BioNTech and Moderna received Emergency Use Authorization (EUA) for the adult vaccines in December 2020, they started recruiting children aged 12–15 for clinical trials. By the summer of 2021, EUA was granted for both vaccines for children 12 years of age and older. By January 2022, Pfizer-BioNTech vaccines were authorized for children aged 5–17. The Centers for Disease Control and Prevention (CDC) recommended COVID-19 vaccines for everyone 5 years of age and older. Boosters were authorized for everyone 12 years of age and older.

Clinical trials for those under the age of 18 created legal issues that vaccine researchers had to address. Anyone who participates in a clinical trial must be given full and complete information. For participants 18 and over, that process is known as informed consent. For those under the age of 18, informed consent is not legally binding. Therefore, researchers use a process adapted to protect the rights of children, known as informed assent. As in adult clinical trials, children or families who wished to withdraw from the trials were allowed to do so.

Vaccination for children against COVID-19 had the same levels of safety and efficacy as adult vaccination. The vaccines were described as a "trifecta" of good news, said one researcher. "We have safety, we got the immune response we wanted—it was actually better than what we saw in the 16- to 25-year-old population—and we had outright demonstration of efficacy" (Hoffman, 2021).

The Facts: The original EUAs for COVID-19 vaccines only applied to adults aged 16 and up in the case of the Pfizer vaccine, and 18 and up in the case of the Moderna vaccine. Children, even teenagers, are not just smaller and younger versions of adults: their immune systems are still developing, just like the rest of their bodies. For that reason, pediatricians—physicians who specialize in the care of patients up to the age of 21—are trained to pay particular attention to physical, mental, and emotional differences between young people and adults, even if they are treated for the same diseases.

Though children were less vulnerable to COVID-19 than adults, it was still a dangerous, and in some cases life-threatening, disease. By May 2021, there were approximately four million known child COVID-19 cases in the United States and approximately 300 deaths. It is likely that there were many more children who were infected but asymptomatic and therefore were not tested. Public health experts expressed particular concern about the virus variants, particularly the Delta variant, which spread more quickly and produced more symptoms in younger people than the original strain. As virus mutations were known to exploit any area of vulnerability in the population, public health officials worried that new mutations might adapt to target younger people.

Pediatricians also expressed deep concern about the mental and emotional health of young people as the pandemic dragged on. Some of the long-term effects of COVID-19 included anxiety and depression, and teenagers are especially vulnerable to both conditions. With schools closed and after-school activities canceled, many children and adolescents reported feeling lonely and isolated. In addition, the economic and emotional turmoil that the pandemic created for many families took a tremendous toll on children as well as parents.

Adults, especially older adults, were at greater risk for serious complications of COVID-19, so it made sense to start by developing a vaccine to protect the more vulnerable part of the population. Concentrating on the adult vaccine also made it possible for working adults to return to jobs, and for businesses and essential services to reopen. By May 2021, over a hundred million U.S. adults had been fully vaccinated. For many parents, the next question after their own vaccination was: When can we vaccinate our children?

From a research point of view, the information gained by vaccinating adults, first as part of clinical trials, and next in real-world settings, provided valuable information about the safety and efficacy of the vaccine. The two doses of vaccine had been found to be 95 percent effective against both the original strain of SARS-CoV-2 and the most prevalent variant. The number of adverse effects from vaccination was vanishingly small compared to the rate of hospitalizations and deaths from the disease.

Among the most valuable research results from adult clinical trials and vaccine administration was the finding that there were no significant differences in vaccine safety or efficacy based on demographic characteristics. That is, there were no significant differences in the vaccination outcomes based on race, gender, or socioeconomic status. Another important research result was that younger people were more likely to experience uncomfortable side effects. Both of these findings were helpful in crafting clinical trials for people aged 12–15. Scientists were especially careful in monitoring side effects for their younger patients. As they expected, younger people were more likely to develop headache and fever as side effects. About 20 percent of the participants aged 12–15 experienced noticeable side effects, as compared to 17 percent among participants aged 16–25. As is common among pediatric patients, though, children were less concerned about them than older adults, and the side effects disappeared rapidly.

The clinical trials in the United States took place in university medical research centers, including Yale University in New Haven, Connecticut; Emory University, partnering with Children's Healthcare in Atlanta, Georgia; and Meharry Medical College in Nashville, Tennessee. Children were recruited for the vaccine trials through schools, pediatricians, and social media. According to trial protocols, participants were told to be careful about posting on social media, in order to protect the privacy of those enrolled. However, many children disregarded this advice, posting on Instagram and TikTok. That, in turn, led to more families applying for the trials.

Depending on how the trials were constructed, either half or two-thirds of the participants were given the vaccine, with the remainder given the placebo. All clinical trials had to adhere to standards of informed assent, meaning that they had to make a special effort to ensure that all participants under the age of 18 were fully informed of all aspects of the study before agreeing to join it. Any forms that they were asked to sign had to be written in clear, age-appropriate language. For example, instead of legal language that might refer to "the study participant" or "the subject," in the third person, assent forms are required to directly address the child as "you." Forms signed by the parent had to use the phrase "your child." That makes it clear to parents and children that they are the ones who will be affected by the trial. Researchers were also required to use age-appropriate forms of communication, including videos, images, and question and answer periods, to make sure that the children fully understood and actively agreed to all the study requirements, including medical procedures, ongoing testing, and their own reporting activities.

Many researchers were happy to be working with younger people, who were often more animated and engaged than adult participants. They showed up on time and were "super compliant." To make sure they knew what was coming, they were asked about their previous experience with injections and side effects. "Do you remember your tetanus shot? Tell me about it," was a typical question, followed by "Here's how this is similar and how it's different." They were asked, too, about whether they were volunteering because they really wanted to, or because their parents told them to. Q&A sessions were especially lively. As one recruiter said, "Usually adults will skim the form, ask a few questions and they're done," she said. "But kids ask way more questions than adults and they're actually listening, which is pretty nice. . . . Of course, they also want to know if the doses will turn them into zombies" (Hoffman, 2021).

Science journalist Sheila Mulroony Eldred wrote about her children's experience as part of the Moderna clinical trial in early 2021. As she explained, it was the first time she and her daughter were excited, not worried, when the 13-year-old developed chills and a slight fever during the trial. "A fever meant she was probably reacting to a real mRNA vaccine, and not a placebo," Eldred wrote. "Maybe she'd won the vaccine lottery!" When her son, aged 16, developed the typical rash on his arm, they were even happier (Eldred, 2021).

The trial was scheduled to last for 13 months, and the teenaged participants had to agree to at least six office visits for checkups, including nasal swabs and blood draws. They also had to keep diaries of their symptoms. The pharmaceuticals provided compensation for participants: $75 per office visit and $30 per week for maintaining the diary. In some trials, parents were compensated for office visits as well, as they had to make sure their children got there. For Eldred's children, the total amount could come to over $1,000, a substantial inducement for compliance (Eldred, 2021).

Many teenaged participants had civic-minded motives for participating in the clinical trials. They saw it as their opportunity to help the world get back to normal, to make it possible for them to see their grandparents and other relatives without worrying about spreading the infection. One 14-year-old participant wrote, "I've been able to go to more places and hang out with my friends more and not like worry so much" (Huertas, 2021). "This is such a blessing we've been given," said another, aged 15. "This is the first thing within the last year that people my age actually have control over. We actually get to do something to make the situation better" (Friedman, 2021). A 12-year-old signed up for the trial "because it would be helping science . . . beat the pandemic. And it was my way of saying thank you to the frontline workers who are keeping us healthy." His 14-year-old sister said, "I thought this would be a really good story I could tell my children and grandchildren— that I tried to help create the vaccine" (Hoffman, 2021).

As people under 18 make up one-third of the U.S. population, the development of safe and effective COVID-19 vaccines was a significant milestone in the fight to stop the spread of the original strain and its variants. COVID-19 vaccines for children were expected to become an important component in the worldwide effort to prevent future pandemics as well.

FURTHER READING

American Academy of Pediatrics and the Children's Hospital Association. 2021. "Children and Covid-19: State Data Report. State Data Report." https://services.aap.org/en/pages/2019-novel-coronavirus-covid-19-infections/children-and-covid-19-state-level-data-report/.

Eldred, Sheila Mulrooney. 2021. "My Teens Are Coronavirus Vaccine Guinea Pigs." *New York Times*. https://www.nytimes.com/2021/02/16/parenting/teen-coronavirus-vaccine-trial.html.

Food and Drug Association (FDA). 2021. "Coronavirus (COVID-19) Update: FDA Authorizes Pfizer-BioNTech COVID-19 Vaccine for Emergency Use in Adolescents in Another Important Action in Fight against Pandemic." https://www.fda.gov/news-events/press-announcements/coronavirus-covid-19-update-fda-authorizes-pfizer-biontech-covid-19-vaccine-emergency-use.

Friedman, Courtney. 2021. "Teen Participant in Moderna Vaccine Trial Pushing for Other Adolescents to Get COVID-19 Shot." *KSAT.* https://www.ksat.com/news/local/2021/05/11/teen-participant-in-moderna-vaccine-trial-pushing-for-other-adolescents-to-get-covid-19-shot/.

Goodnough, Abby, and Jan Hoffman. 2021. "To Vaccinate Younger Teens, States and Cities Look to Schools, Camps, Even Beaches." *New York Times.* https://www.nytimes.com/2021/05/11/health/covid-vaccination-younger-teens.html.

Hoffman, Jan. 2021. "To Get Their Lives Back, Teens Volunteer for Vaccine Trials." *New York Times.* https://www.nytimes.com/2021/02/16/health/covid-vaccine-teens.html.

Huertas, Tiffany. 2021. "Helotes Teen Shares Moderna COVID-19 Vaccine Trial Experience." *KSAT.* https://www.ksat.com/news/local/2021/03/16/helotes-teen-shares-moderna-covid-19-vaccine-trial-experience/.

Macmillan, Carrie. 2021. "Yale Begins Another COVID-19 Vaccine Trial in Children." *Yale Medicine News.* https://www.yalemedicine.org/news/covid-19-vaccine-trial-in-children.

Mandavilli, Apoorva. 2021. "F.D.A. Authorizes Pfizer-BioNTech Vaccine for Children 12 to 15." *New York Times.* https://www.nytimes.com/2021/05/10/health/pfizer-vaccine-children-kids.html.

Q17. WERE SOME COUNTRIES ESPECIALLY EFFECTIVE AT DISTRIBUTING COVID-19 VACCINES?

Answer: Yes. Both Israel and the Republic of Seychelles had very effective early rollouts of COVID-19 vaccines, and both had vaccinated a high percentage of their populations by the spring of 2021. Case studies of both nations show how the science of vaccines interacted with politics, economics, and war.

Though Israel's vaccination rates were very high for the majority of their residents, there was noticeable hesitancy among the country's Orthodox Jewish and Arab communities. Moreover, though vaccination was available to Palestinians who worked in Israeli territory, Israel was criticized for not providing vaccines to the Palestinian communities in the West Bank and Gaza regions. Military conflict broke out in May 2021 between Israel and Palestine, adding to the pressure on the fragile medical infrastructure in Palestinian-controlled territories.

The Republic of Seychelles had the highest vaccination rate in the world through early 2021, and the country reopened for tourism in March

2021. However, a combination of factors, including use of less efficacious vaccines, relaxation of social distancing, and influx of foreign visitors, led to a dangerous spike in COVID-19 cases in May and June.

Though different in many ways, the two countries are similar in having high incomes, effective centralized governments, and robust health care infrastructure. By December 2021, other countries with similar characteristics had achieved even higher vaccination rates. The United Arab Emirates led the world, with 90 percent of its population vaccinated. Singapore, Cambodia, and South Korea had the highest vaccination rates in Asia: 88 percent, 81 percent, and 80 percent, respectively. In Europe, the vaccination leaders included Portugal, Malta, and Spain, with 87 percent, 86 percent, and 80 percent, respectively. In South America, Chile had the highest vaccination rate, at 85 percent.

The Facts: Israel was able to roll out its vaccination program against COVID-19 so effectively for a number of reasons. It is a comparatively small, urbanized country, with a population of approximately 9.3 million in an area the size of New Jersey. As a nation surrounded by hostile Arab countries, it has a high level of integration between its government, emergency management, and health care. Its population is younger than comparable countries in Europe, with an average age of 30 and only 12 percent of the population over 65.

National health insurance is mandatory in Israel, with all citizens required to sign up with one of four not-for-profit health maintenance organizations (HMOs). The four HMOs must provide a certain level of service, and the government provides incentives for them to increase their enrollment. The HMOs thus look for ways to improve their patient services, and Israelis expect high-quality health care delivery and outcomes. They often stay with the same health care providers all their lives—"from cradle to grave"—leading to a high level of trust in doctors and compliance with recommendations for preventative and acute care. As it is a nation frequently at war with its neighbors, Israel also maintains a system of national emergency drills, which include health care disasters. Even before the COVID-19 pandemic, these drills had incorporated the possibility of a national vaccination effort.

The country also has excellent access to digital resources, and its citizens are notably tech-savvy. All children are enrolled in the national vaccination registry, which was easily adapted to COVID-19. Even older people are likely to live near a younger relative who could help them make vaccination appointments online and provide transportation.

All these factors were put into play during the period of vaccine development in 2020. Early on, special funds were allocated to the government to purchase vaccines, and officials kept in close contact with companies as they pursued vaccine research. In the fall of 2020, the Israeli government signed an agreement with Pfizer-BioNTech to obtain some of the earliest shipments of their vaccine, so that they could begin distributing it as soon as it received Emergency Use Authorization from both the World Health Organization (WHO) and its own Ministry of Health.

Israel was able to obtain the early shipment in part because the amount was comparatively small: the nine million doses necessary to vaccinate the entire population could be stored in a single cold-storage facility. With Israel's compact size and transportation infrastructure, vaccine doses could be transported throughout the country from the central storage facility. The Ministry of Health also signed an agreement with Pfizer to provide aggregate patient data regarding the vaccine rollout to Pfizer in a way that protected individual privacy. The country's experience therefore became an excellent real-world test of the safety and efficacy of the vaccine.

Responsibility for vaccinating the Israeli population was efficiently allocated to existing health authorities, starting, as in many countries, with those over 65. Each of the four HMOs was allocated the responsibility for vaccinating their own patients. They had substantial experience in this from former vaccination campaigns, and they were able to use their highly efficient system of community-based nurses for the actual vaccination. Responsibility for vaccinating nursing-home residents was assigned to the national medical emergency services organization.

The number of patients vaccinated began at 8000 per day on December 20, 2020, and nine days later was up to 150,000 per day. According to one report, it took 30 seconds to sign up and five minutes to get each of the two shots. As in other countries, there were public health campaigns and other incentives to persuade Israelis to be vaccinated. Many young people were persuaded by the "green passport," a vaccination certificate allowing them access to gyms, beaches, and restaurants.

Though much of Israel's adult population—close to 60 percent—had been vaccinated by May 2021, certain communities lagged behind. Within the ultra-Orthodox community there was a great deal of hesitancy, based in part on previous distrust of vaccinations and in part on disinformation specific to the COVID-19 vaccine. Arab citizens within Israel were also hesitant to be vaccinated. Members of both communities tended to be lower-income; like low-income and minority groups in other countries, they had less trust in government directives, as well as less access to health care infrastructure.

Israel enforces a blockade against the Palestinian territories of the West Bank and Gaza, regions that have long been a source of military conflict.

In January 2021, independent observers associated with the UN Human Rights Council called on the Israeli government, as an occupying power, to provide COVID-19 vaccines to Palestinians within those territories. Israel disagreed, arguing that though they have an obligation to provide health care to those Palestinians who live, work, and pay taxes within Israel, health care in the two Palestinian territories is the responsibility of their governments. From a human rights perspective this was simply wrong, according to the UN report: "This means that more than 4.5 million Palestinians will remain unprotected and exposed to COVID-19, while Israeli citizens living near and among them—including the Israeli settler population—will be vaccinated. Morally and legally, this differential access to necessary health care in the midst of the worst global health crisis in a century is unacceptable" (UN Human Rights, 2021).

By March, the WHO global vaccine rollout had reached Gaza and the West Bank, with substantial contributions from Arab nations and much smaller ones from Israel. Military conflict between Gaza and Israel in May 2021 overwhelmed the fragile Palestinian health care system and disrupted vaccination efforts. Vaccination efforts only resumed after both sides agreed to a cease-fire.

The vaccine rollout in the Republic of Seychelles began in January 2020, and for several months, it had the welcome reputation of being the most vaccinated nation in the world. The Seychelles are an archipelago of 115 islands in the Indian Ocean. Together with another island nation, Mauritius, it has the highest per capita income in Africa. The local population is only 98,000, but in a normal year, the Seychelles attracts around 350,000 tourists. The tourist industry is key to the economy of the country, employing around 30 percent of the workforce and generating over 70 percent of the gross domestic product (GDP). When the COVID-19 pandemic put a stop to travel, the citizens of the Seychelles were very hard-hit. The Seychelles itself was not devastated by the pandemic. There were under 4,000 cases and only 16 deaths. But tourism plummeted, and as the nation's minister of foreign affairs and tourism reported, "[Since] our economy revolves a lot around tourism, it means that other activities also slowed down. Everything from fishing, to farming, arts and crafts, restaurants and bars. So we started the year in a really bad state" (Hardingham-Gill, 2021).

Once vaccines had been developed, then, the government took immediate steps to obtain them. Half of the nation's supplies consisted of the vaccine known as Sinopharm, developed in China. It contains an inactivated version of SARS-CoV-2, which produced an immune response after only one shot. As it uses the whole virus, it is less fragile than the vaccine produced with mRNA and does not require extremely cold storage. As part of what has been called a campaign of "vaccine diplomacy," China offered Sinopharm free to over 60 countries and entered into commercial agreements with 30 more.

The other half of the vaccination supply in the Seychelles consisted of AstraZeneca vaccines manufactured in India. The AstraZeneca vaccines use DNA to manufacture the protein spike in antigen-presenting cells necessary to produce the immune response. They, too, are less fragile and do not require the extremely cold storage of the Pfizer-BioNTech and Moderna vaccines.

As Sinopharm and the AstraZeneca vaccines are easier to store and ship, they are less expensive to produce, and they have become the vaccines of choice in many parts of the world. But they are less efficacious at producing an immune response than the mRNA vaccines, hovering around the 80 percent effectiveness rate. That means that even fully vaccinated people are at greater risk of developing COVID-19 than people receiving mRNA vaccines, and it also means that they are more likely to spread it.

By March, 61 percent of the population had been vaccinated, and the government decided to take the chance of reopening the country for tourists. It waived almost all requirements for international visitors, as long as they had a negative COVID-19 test up to three days before arrival. The hope was that travel-starved tourists would welcome the opportunity to visit one of the world's most beautiful places. So they did: the number of visitors rose from 708 in February to 4,969 in March and 14,245 in April.

But the number of COVID-19 cases rose as well, with the total caseload surging to over 8,000 (with 32 deaths) by the beginning of May 2021. Approximately 15 percent of the cases were foreign visitors, and 30 percent were locals who had already been vaccinated. Among the already vaccinated who became ill, the cases were milder. But fears that COVID-19 could become widespread throughout the Seychelles' 115 islands led the government to reimpose quarantines and other social distancing regulations.

Although the Seychelles government was criticized for relying on less-effective vaccines, public health experts pointed out that they had behaved much as predicted in the clinical trials. An efficacy rate of around 80 percent means that around 20 percent of those vaccinated may develop COVID-19. A vaccination rate of 61 percent means that 39 percent of the population was not protected at all from the disease. Basic rules of statistics, combined with known behavior of people on vacation—traveling, dining out, going to bars, dancing—meant that a surge in COVID-19 cases in the Republic of the Seychelles was almost inevitable.

As many countries found during the pandemic, it was no easy matter to balance the economic benefits of reopening against the costs of further spreading the disease. The most successful efforts were found in those nations whose political leaders refrained from politicizing the vaccine and instead worked together to build and maintain public trust in science and health care professionals. Public health officials successfully built alliances with local and faith-based communities to overcome vaccine hesitancy and counter misinformation. And there were strong economic incentives to vaccinate as much of the population as quickly as possible to encourage local travel, foreign trade, and tourism.

FURTHER READING

Bariyo, Nicholas. 2021. "Seychelles, the World's Most Vaccinated Nation, Sees Renewed Covid-19 Surge." *Wall Street Journal.* https://www.wsj .com/articles/seychelles-the-worlds-most-vaccinated-nation -sees-renewed-covid-19-surge-11620669853.

Cunningham, Erin. 2021. "Israel's Military Assault on Gaza Threatens to Worsen the Pandemic in the Enclave." *Washington Post.* https://www .washingtonpost.com/world/israel-gaza-hamas-coronavirus -pandemic/2021/05/13/0a2e571a-b310-11eb-bc96-fdf55de43bef_story.html.

Hardingham-Gill, Tamara. 2021. "How the Seychelles Is Racing to Become the World's Safest Destination." *CNN Travel.* https://www.cnn.com /travel/article/seychelles-reopens-to-travelers/index.html.

Holder, Josh. 2021. "Tracking Coronavirus Vaccinations around the World." *New York Times.* https://www.nytimes.com/interactive/2021/world /covid-vaccinations-tracker.html.

Hollingsworth, Julia. 2021. "The Seychelles Is 60% Vaccinated, but Still Infections Are Rising. That's Not as Bad as It Sounds." *CNN.* https:// www.cnn.com/2021/05/14/africa/seychelles-covid-vaccination-infection -intl-hnk-dst/index.html.

Republic of the Seychelles. National Bureau of Statistics. 2021. *Statistical Bulletin.* "Visitor Arrivals April 2021." Released May 7, 2021. https:// www.nbs.gov.sc/68nn-5292-8nn-27622-nnhi/.

Rosen, Bruce, Sarah Dine, and Nadav Davidovitch. 2021. "Lessons in COVID-19 Vaccination from Israel." *Health Affairs.* https://www .healthaffairs.org/do/10.1377/hblog20210315.476220/full/.

Rosen, Bruce, Ruth Waitzberg, and Avi Israeli. 2021. "Israel's Rapid Rollout of Vaccinations for COVID-19." *Israeli Journal of Health Policy Research* 10 (6). https://doi.org/10.1186/s13584-021-00440-6.

Schwartz, Felicia, and Yaroslav Trofimov. 2021. "How Israel Delivered the World's Fastest Vaccine Rollout." *Wall Street Journal.* https://www.wsj .com/articles/how-israel-delivered-the-worlds-fastest-vaccine-rollout -11616080968.

United Nations Human Rights. Office of the High Commissioner. 2021.
"Israel/OPT: UN Experts Call on Israel to Ensure Equal Access to COVID-
19 Vaccines for Palestinians." https://www.ohchr.org/EN/NewsEvents
/Pages/DisplayNews.aspx?NewsID=26655.

Q18. DID SOME COUNTRIES FACE MAJOR CHALLENGES IN DISTRIBUTING COVID-19 VACCINES?

Answer: Yes. India experienced significant challenges in its COVID-19
vaccine rollout. India is the second most populated country in the world
(after China), with 1.38 billion people. That alone made it especially vulnerable to infectious disease, and public health officials expected vaccination to play a key role in controlling COVID-19. The complex tasks
involved in manufacturing, shipping, and administering billions of doses
required careful planning.

To put the numbers into context, India routinely vaccinates 55 million
people per year. To vaccinate everyone against COVID-19, public health
officials would have to administer 25 times that number of shots. Even if
officials took as their goal the 60 percent vaccination rate achieved by
Israel and the Republic of the Seychelles that meant vaccinating 858 million people, more than 15 times the usual number. National and state
preparation for such a massive upscale in vaccination efforts began early in
the pandemic, as it did elsewhere in the world.

Initially, there was good reason for optimism. India is the largest pro-
ducer of vaccines in the world. One company, the Serum Institute of
India, estimates that two-thirds of children around the globe are vaccinated with their products. By September 2020, the Serum Institute had
signed an agreement with Oxford-AstraZeneca to manufacture one billion doses of the vaccine, marketed in India as Covishield. Half would be
reserved for India, and the other half would be made available for global
initiatives providing COVID-19 vaccines to low-income countries. By
early 2021, two other vaccines were approved for use in India. Collec-
tively, the three types of vaccines were expected to provide enough doses
to protect the population.

Moreover, public health officials had taken steps to strengthen India's
already-effective vaccination infrastructure by training additional health
care workers in both urban and rural areas. They planned for additional
cold storage facilities and security personnel to make sure that vaccine
shipments could be safely transported and stored throughout the country.

Unfortunately, the start of the India's vaccine rollout coincided with a devastating second wave of the pandemic. At its peak, there were 400,000 new cases and more than 4,000 deaths reported each day. Medical centers and other facilities were overwhelmed, and medical personnel turned their attention to acute care instead of administering vaccines. Vaccine manufacturers, already working at peak capacity, had no way to scale up production to meet the new demand.

As the number of cases surged, foreign governments, international agencies, and private companies sent money, therapeutics, raw materials, and extra vaccine doses to India. At the same time, Indian public health officials worked hard to vaccinate the most vulnerable members of the population, end the second wave, and prevent any future surges.

The Facts: India was hard-hit by the first wave of the COVID-19 pandemic, which began in that country in January 2020 and peaked in September 2020. The seven-day average of the daily caseload—a measure used by many virus trackers to limit fluctuations caused by inconsistencies in report—reached over 93,000 new cases per day at its height. The caseload had been doubling every month. Moreover, in its peak, there were over 1,000 deaths per day.

National, state, and municipal governments imposed stringent lockdowns, and the caseload eased. By February 2021, the seven-day average of new COVID-19 cases was down to around 12,000 per day, with around 100 deaths per day. There were occasional flare-ups attributed to mass gatherings, including important religious festivals that attracted thousands of people. Still, during the early months of 2021, there was a great deal of optimism that the pandemic in India might have burnt itself out, infecting enough people so that the vaccines, once administered, would quickly lead to population immunity.

Certainly, there was every reason to think that India could produce enough vaccines for its own population as well as those abroad. India has been a world leader in vaccine production for many years, with excellent resources for scientific development, for cold storage, and for distribution. The logistics of trying to import vaccines from other countries would be impossible for such a large and well-populated nation, requiring thousands of flights in specially designed airplanes.

In order to ensure vaccine supply, the Serum Institute of India signed contracts with several companies developing the new vaccines. Their investment paid off with AstraZeneca, marketed in India as Covishield. The company began manufacturing in the fall of 2020, and it had stockpiled 50 million doses by the start of India's vaccine rollout in January

2021. The vaccine manufacturer was able to boost production to 70 million doses per month through the spring of 2021 and planned on increasing production still further over the summer to reach its goal of one billion doses by the end of 2021.

Another Indian pharmaceutical company, Bharat Biotech International Ltd., developed and tested the vaccine Covaxin, produced with an inactivated form of SARS-CoV-2. Approximately 150 million doses were scheduled to be produced by the summer of 2021, with 500 million by the end of the year. Both the Serum Institute and Bharat Biotech also began production of newer vaccines that were expected to be approved for emergency use by the fall of 2021. Other companies began production of Sputnik V, a COVID-19 vaccine developed by the National Center of Epidemiology and Microbiology of Moscow. A goal of half a billion doses of the vaccines by the end of 2021 seemed feasible.

Of course, half a billion doses would only vaccinate about a third of the country's population. But as in all countries, public health officials counted on getting the vaccine to the most vulnerable members of the population first—health care workers, older people, and those with preexisting medical conditions. As long as the case rate remained low, officials thought, they had time to distribute the vaccines as they became available.

However, in early February 2021, the caseload started to rise, first to 11,000 patients per day, and then to 22,000, and then to 90,000. By the end of April, the seven-day average was up over 300,000 cases per day, with a death rate of over 4000 per day. In some communities, the percentage of people who tested positive was over 30 percent, meaning that one in three people had the disease. Hospitals were flooded with patients, and critical care units, especially, were overwhelmed. Public health officials turned sports halls, stadiums, and ashrams into COVID-19 hospitals. Railway cars were turned into 12-bed treatment facilities, named COVID Care Centers. Oxygen, especially, was in short supply, and officials created Oxygen Express routes on major rail lines to deliver oxygen to cities that had become epicenters of the second wave. The Indian Air Force and commercial airlines flew in oxygen from countries that could spare it, from Singapore to the United States and Canada.

There were three key reasons for the rapid uptick in India's caseload. The first was the spread of new variants. The Alpha variant, B.1.1.7, had reached India by early 2021; though not associated with a higher death rate than the original strain, it is more infectious and is as likely to cause respiratory distress. The Delta variant, B.1.617.2, was identified in the state of Maharashtra in March 2021. It, too, spreads more rapidly than the original strain, and by April it accounted for more than half of India's new cases.

By December 2021, Omicron, B.1.1.529 had been identified in India, and by January 2022, it was the dominant strain.

A second reason the cases of COVID-19 skyrocketed was the relaxation of social distancing restrictions and mask wearing. By February 2021, in India as around the globe, people were fed up with pandemic-based restrictions on normal life. The rapid drop in India's caseload after its first wave made many people think that the worst was over. A religious festival that attracted 55 million people in early April 2021 led to more than 2,000 new COVID-19 cases. Large political rallies also helped spread the disease. In India as elsewhere, new lockdowns were highly unpopular, as there was widespread concern about compounding the health care crisis with an economic crisis that could leave many people vulnerable to hunger and homelessness.

A third reason for the surge in COVID-19 cases in India was the lack of additional resources for the already-overworked health care system, combined with the pace of the vaccine rollout. By May 2021, India had vaccinated approximately 191 million people. This was a substantial achievement, especially for a country with a health care system in a state of crisis. To put this figure in perspective, it is 19 times the number of doses administered in Israel at the same period, and roughly two-thirds of the number of doses administered in the United States. The difference is in the total population: 191 million vaccinated people form only 14 percent of the Indian population.

As nearly half the new cases were in rural districts, public health officials worked closely with local communities to convince as many people as possible to be vaccinated. An important part of the process was listening to local communities to understand the reasons they might be hesitant. In one village, residents were fearful that the new vaccines might be dangerous: to combat that fear, village leaders agreed to be vaccinated and to go door-to-door to speak to residents. Some residents were also fearful that if they agreed to be tested for COVID-19, they would be sent away to distant hospitals away from family. To combat that fear, community health officials converted local schools to COVID-19 treatment centers. They also held a vaccination camp in conjunction with a local religious celebration. As the number of vaccinated people increased, fewer and fewer people were hesitant. In India, as elsewhere, local leadership and local community support were key to successful vaccination. By February 2022, 55% of the population—over 760 million people—were fully vaccinated.

India's health care crisis had an international ripple effect. The soaring caseload created even greater demand for COVID-19 vaccines, so the government suspended their export outside of India. That meant that people in lower-income nations who had been depending on shipments of vaccines manufactured in India faced devastating shortages. By the winter of 2022, as high vaccination rates led wealthier nations to look forward to the end of the pandemic, low-income nations confronted ongoing health care crises without the vaccine doses necessary to fully protect their population.

FURTHER READING

Bendix, Aria. 2021. "A Perfect Storm of 4 Factors Has Fueled India's Harrowing Coronavirus Surge. Other Countries Could Be Next." *Business Insider.* https://www.businessinsider.com/india-coronavirus-cases-deaths-lesson-stay-alert-2021-4.

Changoiwala, Puja. 2021. "How a Village in India Reached 100% Vaccination in the Face of Misinformation and Hesitancy." *National Geographic.* https://www.nationalgeographic.com/science/article/how-a-village-in-india-reached-100-vaccination-in-the-face-of-misinformation-and-hesitancy.

"Covid-19 in India: Cases, Deaths and Oxygen Supply." 2021. *BBC.* https://www.bbc.com/news/world-asia-india-56891016.

Kumar, Velayudhan Mohan, Seithikurippu R. Pandi-Perumal, Ilya Trakht, and Sadras Panchatcharam Thyagarajan. 2021. "Strategy for COVID-19 Vaccination in India: The Country with the Second Highest Population and Number of Cases." *NPJ Vaccines* 6 (60). https://doi.org/10.1038/s41541-021-00327-2.

The Lancet Covid-19 Commission, India Task Force. 2021. *Country-wide Containment Strategies for Reducing COVID-19 Cases in India.* https://static1.squarespace.com/static/5ef3652ab722df11fcb2ba5d/t/60a3cf08d1c1f24480a44c19/1621348107249/India+TF+Country-wide+Containment+Strategies+April+2021.pdf.

Mullick, Jamie. 2020. "India's First Covid Wave Finally Recedes." *Hindustan Times.* https://www.hindustantimes.com/india-news/india-s-first-covid-19-wave-finally-recedes/story-clQaMmmD2TiYD3i1CSmw3J.html.

Schmall, Emily and Karen Deep Singh. 2021. "Amid Second Covid Wave, World Responds to India's Distress Call." *New York Times.* https://www.nytimes.com/2021/04/26/world/asia/india-covid-vaccine-world-response.html.

Yasir, Sameer, Shashank Bengali, and Rick Gladstone. 2021. "Mass Vaccination, India's Covid-19 Escape Route, Poses a Giant Challenge." *New York Times.* https://www.nytimes.com/2021/04/29/world/asia/india-coronavirus-vaccines.html.

Q19. WERE GLOBAL EFFORTS UNDERTAKEN TO EFFECTIVELY DISTRIBUTE COVID-19 VACCINES THROUGHOUT THE WORLD?

Answer: Yes. In April 2020, the World Health Organization (WHO) partnered with government officials, private organizations, and UNICEF (United Nations Children's Fund) to create a working group called the Access to COVID-19 Tools (ACT) Accelerator. The ACT Accelerator had two goals: (1) rapid development of vaccines and tools for treating for COVID-19 and (2) equitable and global access to vaccines and other resources. The COVID-19 vaccine division of the ACT Accelerator was named COVAX.

COVAX's main objective was to do for the rest of the world what wealthy nations were already doing for their own residents: prepurchase huge quantities of vaccine doses from the manufacturers as they were developed and approved. They could then be distributed at minimal cost to low-income countries that could not afford to purchase their own vaccine supplies. They could also be supplied to middle-income countries that might be able to afford some number of vaccines, but would have a hard time competing on an open global market for scarce vaccine supplies. Funding came originally from the wealthier European nations and Canada. The United States joined the effort as the largest donor in January 2021 with the incoming Biden administration. Philanthropies with a long history of supporting global vaccination efforts, including the Bill and Melinda Gates Foundation, provided both financial support and technical expertise.

The logistics side of COVAX is handled by UNICEF, as a natural outgrowth of the organization's pre-COVID-19 role as the leading vaccinator of the world's children. Every year, UNICEF manages the vaccination of over two billion children for all the major childhood diseases, such as diphtheria, measles, and polio. They also arrange for the production and distribution of vaccines to people of all ages in cases of emergency outbreaks, such as Ebola. As Ann Ottosen, senior manager with UNICEF's supply division, put it, "Our job is to secure the right vaccines, in the right quantities at the right time" (UNICEF, "COVAX: 'We have achieved,'" 2021).

Many people and governments see equitable distribution of COVID-19 vaccines around the world as a moral imperative. It also makes good economic sense for the wealthy countries who are providing most of the funding. Wealthy countries do not exist on their own. Vital components of manufacturing in the world's most resilient economies—Canada, France, Germany, Japan, Qatar, South Korea, Sweden, United Arab Emirates, United Kingdom and the United States—rely on raw materials and other resources supplied by people in lower-income nations. They are vital links in the global supply chain. If they continue to be ravaged by COVID-19, they will not suffer alone: instead, at least half of the total economic loss—perhaps amounting to as much as $9 trillion—will be borne by their more industrialized trading partners.

As one economist put it, "No economy will be fully recovered unless the other economies are recovered" (Goodman, 2021). Tedros Adhanom Ghebreyesus, director-general of WHO, stated even more bluntly the message from COVID-19 to the postpandemic world: "None of us is safe until all of us are safe" (WHO, 2021).

The Facts: When stakeholders met in April 2020 to establish the ACT Accelerator, they had a clear example of what *not* to do in a global pandemic. It came from the experience of the H1N1 pandemic in 2009–10, which infected an estimated 60 million people in the United States. The outbreak was first reported in the United States in April 2009, and by October, several pharmaceutical companies had developed candidate vaccines. At the time, vaccine researchers were widely praised for their ability to meet the pandemic threat in such a timely fashion. After its initial distribution, the H1N1 vaccine was incorporated into seasonal influenza vaccines in subsequent years.

The problem was that access to the H1N1 vaccines was almost entirely limited to wealthy nations who could afford to purchase them in bulk from pharmaceutical companies. There was no provision whatsoever for timely distribution of the vaccine to the rest of the world. Even if money had been available for UNICEF to purchase H1N1 vaccines, the fact that these were brand-new vaccines meant that supplies were limited. Wealthy nations, including the United States, acted like supermarket shoppers in the early days of COVID-19 lockdowns: they bought up all available supplies, including medical equipment, treatment, and vaccines, and stockpiled them for their own country's use. By the time money had been allocated to global public health organizations for H1N1 vaccine purchases elsewhere in the world, very limited supplies were left.

This scenario is often referred to as "vaccine nationalism," in which each nation looks after its own, narrowly defined interest instead of considering the common interests of all nations. Such an outcome for the COVID-19 pandemic would have been disastrous. The SARS-CoV-2 virus was much more deadly and infectious than H1N1, and within six months, it had developed a set of mutations of concern. As it spread worldwide, health experts issued prescient warnings that the disease would develop mutations, also known as variants, that could undermine the effectiveness of the first round of vaccines. The global cost, in both unnecessary deaths and economic losses, would not be limited to vaccine-have-not nations and individuals. It would have a profound impact on vaccine-haves as well.

The original goal set by COVAX was to distribute 2.5 billion doses by the end of 2021. That would have been enough to vaccinate 20 percent of the world, with priority to go to health care professionals. Though that would not be nearly enough to stop the spread of COVID-19, it would be enough to ensure that frontline health care workers were protected globally. Some participants would have liked "vaccine-have" governments to pledge that COVID-19 vaccines be made available for 20 percent of the entire world before they stockpiled vaccines for the remaining 80 percent of their own populations. Sadly, that was never likely to happen. The governments of the world's wealthiest nations had strong incentives to purchase enough vaccines for their own populations first, before donating either money or unused vaccines to the rest of the globe.

By October 2021, COVAX had nonetheless distributed over 400 million vaccine doses. It also projected a distribution of 1.4 billion doses by the end of 2021. How did it manage this daunting logistical feat? Even before the first vaccine was approved for emergency use, UNICEF began working on the necessary infrastructure for a program of global vaccination. Public health and procurement officials from each participating country worked closely with UNICEF personnel who had many years of experience with their country's needs. All 189 of the recipient countries—92 low-income and 97 middle-income countries—developed distribution plans to make sure that vaccines, when they arrived, would be transported to people as soon as possible. They also agreed to abide by WHO instructions on the importance of a phased rollout, so that those most in danger of infection and death would get the vaccine shipments first. At the top of the list are frontline health care professionals as well as support staff in health care settings. Next are people over 65, as they have had the most severe reactions to COVID-19 infections. And third are people under 65 with underlying health conditions that make them especially vulnerable.

For full transparency, UNICEF published toolkits to help countries prepare. These provided guidance on how to inform their country's population about the vaccine; how to set up, monitor, and protect transportation and cold-storage facilities; how to organize and then track vaccine shipments from port of entry to their distribution centers; how to dispose of medical waste safely, being sure to protect the environment as well as people; and how to maintain all the necessary data for tracking vaccine impact as well as side effects.

All the planning paid off on February 15, 2021, when WHO authorized the AstraZeneca vaccine. As it only required one dose, it was considered the most efficient option for the first round of global vaccines. The UNI-CEF supply group immediately notified their manufacturing partner, Serum Institute of India, to ready the first set of 600,000 doses for ship-ment to Ghana, the country selected to be the first recipient. "The amount of coordination required to fast track the shipments was a huge challenge," remembered Mounir Bouazar, the logistics lead in UNICEF's supply divi-sion. "The vaccines were ready in Mumbai and the syringes were in our hub in Dubai—and we had a window of two to three days to make the delivery happen. In the end, we managed to send a flight from Shanghai to Dubai which was diverted to Mumbai exceptionally for UNICEF to pick up the vaccines. It then stopped over in Dubai to uplift the syringes before loading vaccines and syringes on another flight to Ghana." This was all accomplished within 72 hours, which one of the managers of the supply effort described as "a great achievement. The supplier fast-tracked their timelines, the airlines came up with a solution, and the freight forwarder even donated the flight for free to UNICEF" ("COVAX: Probably the Most Complex Logistical Challenge," 2021).

The doses arrived in Ghana on February 24, 2021. They were deployed across the country, going first to health care professionals. In a country where critical care and oxygen supplies are limited, the vaccines provided an enormous ray of hope. One physician in Accra, the capital of Ghana, explained that he had already seen too many COVID-19 victims die, including his own sister. "I know what COVID has cost," he said, "socially, economically and in the loss of life." Despite side effects, he regarded his own vaccination as "a great experience" (Prabhu, 2021).

By the beginning of April, COVAX had delivered 38 million doses to 100 countries across six continents. Operations in many of these countries posed their own unique challenges. In the mountainous South Asian nation of Nepal, for example, UNICEF had been working for years to set up a network of cold storage units that do not rely on electricity. Between 2020 and 2021, an additional 1,000 cold storage units were established across the country. After the COVID-19 vaccines arrived at the interna-tional airport in Kathmandu, they were transported onward by air, road, and, finally, by porter to reach the most remote regions. In the Sudan, 800,000 doses of the AstraZeneca vaccine and 4.5 tons of syringes had arrived by March. In addition to the usual logistics challenges, vaccine hesitancy was also widespread. Local community groups who had worked on previous vaccination campaigns provided outreach and support to ensure that the vaccine was available to the most vulnerable populations.

The devastating second wave of COVID-19 infections in India inter-rupted the global rollout of COVID-19 vaccines. The majority of COVAX's advance purchase agreements were with Indian pharmaceutical companies, and as the COVID-19 crisis in India worsened, companies were hard pressed to keep up with both the domestic and international demand. COVAX leaders and their many international partners called on vaccine-have nations and on pharmaceutical companies worldwide to provide funding, manufacturing capacity, and available vaccine doses to support the global vaccination effort. By February 2022, COVAX had shipped over 1 billion doses of COVID-19 vaccines to 144 jurisdictions.

In the modern world, where infectious disease is only a plane ride away, public health authorities assert that it is the responsibility of vaccine-rich communities to ensure that vaccines are only a plane ride away as well.

FURTHER READING

Beaubien, Jason. 2021. "What Is This COVAX Program That the U.S. Is Pouring Millions of Vaccines Into?" *National Public Radio (NPR)*. https://www.npr.org/sections/goatsandsoda/2021/05/19/998228372/what-is-this-covax-program-that-the-u-s-is-pouring-millions-of-vaccines-into.

Berkley, Seth. 2021. "The World Isn't Getting Vaccinated Fast Enough. Here Are 4 Ways to Fix That." *Time*. https://time.com/6047516/covax-covid-19-vaccine-access/.

Goodman, Peter. 2021. "If Poor Countries Go Unvaccinated, a Study Says, Rich Ones Will Pay." *New York Times*. https://www.nytimes.com/2021/01/23/business/coronavirus-vaccines-global-economy.html.

Prabhu, Maya. 2021. "'We'll All Be Fine': COVID-19 Vaccines Arrive at Korle-Bu Teaching Hospital, Accra." *GAVI—The Vaccine Alliance*. https://www.gavi.org/vaccineswork//well-all-be-fine-covid-19-vaccines-arrive-korle-bu-teaching-hospital-accra.

United Nations International Children's Emergency Fund (UNICEF). n.d. "COVAX: Probably the Most Complex Logistical Challenge in History." Accessed May 29, 2021. https://www.unicef.org/supply/covax-probably-most-complex-logistical-challenge-history.

United Nations International Children's Emergency Fund (UNICEF). n.d. "COVAX: We Have Achieved Something That Has Never Been Done Before." Accessed May 29, 2021. https://www.unicef.org/supply/covax-we-have-achieved-something-has-never-been-done.

United Nations International Children's Emergency Fund (UNICEF). n.d. "Reaching the Unreached: COVID-19 Vaccinations in Jumla." Accessed May 29, 2021. https://www.unicef.org/nepal/stories/reaching-unreached-covid-19-vaccinations-jumla.

World Health Organization (WHO). 2021. *ACT Now, ACT Together. 2020–2021 Impact Report.* https://www.who.int/publications/m/item/act-now-act-together-2020-2021-impact-report.

World Health Organization (WHO). 2020. COVAX: *The Vaccines Pillar of the Access to Covid-19 Tools (ACT) Accelerator. Structure and Principles.* https://www.who.int/publications/m/item/covax-the-vaccines-pillar-of-the-access-to-covid-19-tools-(act)-accelerator.

3

❖❖❖

Key Issues in Global Vaccination

INTRODUCTION

This section explores the role of vaccination in preventing global outbreaks of disease. What do vaccines and vaccination programs look like from a global perspective? How are they distributed around the world, and what are the barriers to equitable distribution? What are the roles of international and national public health agencies, of governmental regulatory bodies, and of philanthropies in manufacturing and distributing safe and effective vaccines? What are the ongoing factors that can disrupt vaccine supply chains, including armed conflict and crime? And what are the global efforts to promote accurate vaccine information and advocacy, so that worldwide vaccination programs can save the lives of more people?

Throughout human history, what began as small outbreaks of infectious diseases have become epidemics and pandemics, spreading from person to person and community to community. This phenomenon was well known in the earliest human societies. Some of the earliest mechanisms for dealing with it include quarantine of people and goods, preventing them from entering a community until a specific period of time—originally, 40 days—had passed, when the dangers of any infection they might carry was likely to be over. Another way of dealing with infection involved the provision of hospitals for people with infectious diseases, where they could be cared for without risk of their passing the disease on to their families or neighbors. In extreme cases, such as outbreaks of the bubonic plague or Ebola, lockdowns could be placed on entire communities, preventing people and goods from entering or leaving.

As we now know, many pathogens can mutate and adapt to human societies much faster than human laws and customs can adapt to them. Quarantines, hospitals, and lockdowns have historically slowed, but not stopped, the spread of infectious diseases. This occurs not only because of the biology of disease organizations but also because of the ingenuity of their human hosts at evading regulations. Individuals have always put their own views on the best way to protect themselves and their families ahead of even the best-intentioned regulations designed to restrict their movements. Some of the most graphic accounts we have of the bubonic plague in Europe are of those who attempted to flee from the disease, only to take it with them to supposedly safe communities.

The bubonic plague moved around the world in the 14th century primarily by following the movements of people and goods. At that time the world's population has been estimated at about 400 million people. Now, it is estimated at 7,875 billion people, and our transportation networks extend to every corner of the globe. They were designed to move people and goods as quickly and efficiently as possible from remote rural villages to large manufacturing cities and back again. They have proved, time and time again, to be enormously quick and efficient at spreading diseases as well.

For that reason, the modern global world could not survive without modern global vaccination policies and programs. Smallpox vaccination practices have been fairly widespread since the beginning of the 19th century, but in the century before its eradication in 1980, the disease is estimated to have killed about 500 million people. Since 1980, the incidence of cases and deaths from vaccine-preventable diseases has declined by 80 percent.

In the case of COVID-19, we know from data compiled as of November 2021 that vaccinated people are one-sixth as likely to test positive as those who are not vaccinated. If they do test positive, they are approximately one-third as likely to transmit it. Based on that data, many countries that had placed restrictions on international travel took steps to end them for fully vaccinated people.

Though global vaccination programs and policies undoubtedly made the world a safer, healthier place, it could not erase long-standing inequities in health care practices. For much of the world's history, access to health care, including vaccines, was treated as any other consumer good, with wealthy people having greater access and choice than poor people. Wealthy countries with stable health care systems can advise—and, in some circumstances, require—as many as 27 different types of vaccines for their residents. These vaccines provide protection from dangerous infectious diseases from cradle to the grave, including childhood diseases, seasonal influenza, workplace-specific diseases such as rabies, and diseases such as shingles that disproportionately affect seniors. In wealthy developed nations, vaccines are often available in multiple convenient locations, including doctor's offices, urgent care facilities, pharmacy chains, and workplace clinics. In cases of outbreaks, pop-up vaccination clinics can be set up in schools, community centers, and malls.

In contrast, vaccination opportunities for residents in low- to middle-income countries are much more circumscribed. Children in many parts of the world may only have access to the vaccines for diphtheria, tetanus, and pertussis (DTaP), and even then only if their health care system is stable enough for them to receive the initial shot and two boosters. Adults may have access to rabies vaccines only in emergencies, and they may have no access to vaccines that could protect them against seasonal influenza or other preventable infections. By December 2021, adults in many countries were still awaiting access to COVID-19 vaccines that were widely available in wealthy countries six months earlier.

The existing income disparities in global vaccine distribution are only made worse by circumstances that affect political and social stability, such as outbreaks of armed conflict, fraud, and crime. Areas of the world with fragile or underfunded health care systems may also have unstable governments or be enmeshed in civil and social conflict. International organizations that work directly with such areas have made it a priority to negotiate to keep health care facilities as neutral ground and to continue vaccination programs whenever possible.

Many international experts believe that the 21st century will mark a decisive change in global policies toward vaccine-preventable disease. They believe there will be more coordination in tracking and preventing vaccine-preventable epidemics before they spread and in funding research that will provide a strong basis for creating new vaccines when new pathogens appear. Philanthropic foundations and international financial institutions such as the World Bank have developed mechanisms to make vaccine manufacture and delivery cost-effective for lower- to middle-income nations. The questions in this section, therefore, highlight obstacles—and potential ways forward—in making future pandemics less threatening for *all* peoples and nations.

Q20. ARE VACCINATION EFFORTS MORE EFFECTIVE IN SOME PARTS OF THE WORLD THAN OTHERS?

Answer: Yes. In general, differences in the extent and effectiveness of vaccination campaigns run along wealth lines, with most people, especially children, having access to far more vaccines in wealthy countries than in poor ones. Even within wealthy countries, there is often a vaccine gap that echoes the wealth gap, with the wealthiest 20 percent in some countries enjoying much greater access to far more vaccines than the poorest 20 percent.

For most vaccines, their actual effectiveness does not depend on wealth. For example, the diphtheria, pertussis, and tetanus (DPT, or DTaP) vaccine protects children equally, whether the children are rich or poor, or living in high-income or low-income countries. But the rotavirus vaccine, which protects against a virus that causes diarrhea, vomiting, and severe dehydration, has been shown to be more effective for children in wealthier countries than in poorer countries.

Different regions of the world also have different needs and priorities with respect to vaccination. DPT vaccines are considered the most basic component of child immunization policies, and their distribution is widely used as a key metric for vaccination coverage in a specific region. But some vaccines, like those against yellow fever and malaria, are only routinely administered in regions where they are endemic. Vaccines intended to stop an outbreak, like those for Ebola, are only administered when outbreaks occur.

Worldwide, there have been significant improvements in vaccination over the past 40 years. In 1990, 5.5 million children died of vaccine-preventable diseases. By 2017, that number had decreased to 1.8 million deaths (Vanderslott, 2019).

The Facts: In countries throughout the world, people strongly support vaccination for children. The global average of support is 92 percent, or 9 out of every 10 people. However, studies have found a north-south divide: support is highest, well over 90 percent in Southeast Asia, South America, and Africa. It is lowest, though still between 80 percent and 90 percent, in North America and Europe. Roughly speaking, the divide marks differences in direct experience of serious vaccine-preventable disease. In regions where vaccine-preventable infections are still endemic, and vaccines are most necessary to prevent against serious illness and death, just about everyone wants their children to have them. In regions where many people are so fortunate as to seldom encounter vaccine-preventable disease, parents may not always realize the role vaccines can play in protecting their children.

Vaccination has long been a priority for the World Health Organization (WHO). WHO, founded in 1948, is a specialized agency within the United Nations, maintaining six regional offices and 150 regional offices. Its chief objective is the "attainment by all peoples of the highest possible level of health" (WHO, *Basic Documents* 2020). It does this by working with its 194 member nations to strengthen infrastructure, promote scientific research and health communication, and develop mechanisms for equitable distribution of health care resources. Particularly in the past 25 years, WHO has focused on the importance of equal access, among all nations, to the opportunities for long life and well-being once limited to the wealthiest individuals of the wealthy nations. As the website states, "Dedicated to the well-being of all people and guided by science, the World Health Organization leads and champions global efforts to give everyone, everywhere an equal chance to live a healthy life" (About WHO, accessed June 22, 2021).

WHO's six regions of operations are Africa, the Americas, South-East Asia, Europe, Eastern Mediterranean, and Western Pacific While all share common goals, specific health care policies and projects are set by the individual regions, depending on the needs of their member countries. The African region, for example, has seen notable gains in recent years. The most visible advance was the successful development of a vaccine for Ebola, long feared for its high mortality rate and lack of treatment options. Vaccines have been successfully introduced against other widespread pathogens as well, such as malaria and cholera. However, the African region remains severely limited in facilities for research, development, and production of innovative and region-specific vaccines. Many African countries lack effective government support for medical research, which is both expensive in its own right and requires additional funding for regulatory bodies and public health facilities. Private sector funding for vaccine manufacturing is often not an option either. And many countries face a severe shortage of trained scientists with the expertise necessary to carry out research.

For these reasons, the African region is dependent on vaccines produced elsewhere in the world and then made available for purchase. One result is that in any global health care crisis, African nations are at the mercy of vaccine-producing nations as to when supplies will arrive. This occurred with the COVID-19 vaccines, when a devasting spike in cases in India led to major delays in shipments intended for Africa. Another result is that diseases that are of major importance in Africa, but not as much of a health burden elsewhere, may be seen as a low priority for vaccine research. If the African region could develop additional vaccine research and production capabilities, it would be less dependent on external supply and demand.

Other regions have set additional priorities. Countries in the Western Pacific region have historically high levels of government support and private funding for health care infrastructure and vaccination research, development, and production. Goals for the region in the recent past have focused on eliminating measles and rubella. Both are highly infectious diseases, and even a small percentage of unvaccinated people may provide opportunities for the pathogens to spread to vulnerable populations. The Americas region comprises enormous extremes of wealth and poverty, and its vaccination goals are accordingly wide-ranging. "The Region of the Americas has one of the highest vaccine coverage levels in the world," according to its director. "However, in spite of this, many hard-to-reach populations are left behind" (PAHO, WHO, "Immunization," 2021).

For example, Tarija, a district in Bolivia, has one of the highest incidents of cervical cancer, amounting to three out of every 100 women. The human papillomavirus (HPV) vaccine has been shown to reduce the prevalence of cervical cancer, and it was routinely given to young girls in schools in Tarija. The COVID-19 pandemic disrupted the usual administration of all vaccines as well as other routine health care. Once conditions eased, medical staff from urban areas in the district made it a priority to travel to remote rural regions to administer the two required doses of the HPV vaccines that protect women from cancer.

Nearly all vaccines currently administered have the same success rate across all regions. For example, a DTaP or measles vaccine will be just as efficacious in one region or country as in another. The rotavirus vaccines are an exception to this rule, however. Rotavirus infections attack the gastrointestinal tract, leading to diarrhea, vomiting, and dehydration. They are treatable, but the treatments are costly, and may include intravenous delivery of fluids and medication. Children under the age of five are most vulnerable, and those living in areas without easy access to abundant, treated water are especially so. Over 500,000 children die from rotavirus infection each year, and over 95 percent of the victims are from low-income countries.

In 2009, WHO added the rotavirus vaccine to its list of recommended childhood vaccines, and the public-private partnership GAVI, the Global Vaccine Alliance, provided funding to introduce it to low-income countries. Studies in Asia and Africa showed that introduction of rotavirus vaccines were effective in preventing severe rotavirus disease in children under one year of age.

Subsequent studies showed, however, that the vaccines were more effective in preventing severe rotavirus disease in high-income countries with lower childhood mortality than in low-income countries with high childhood mortality. Scientists have not been able to pinpoint why it should be less effective in poorer countries, but some have suggested that poor overall nutrition and exposure to more sources of the virus might be significant factors.

Since lack of access to vaccines is so closely associated with low-income countries and regions, WHO, GAVI, and other organizations have worked closely with the United Nations Children's Fund (UNICEF) to provide vaccines. The name "UNICEF" comes from the initials of the earliest version of the organization, the United Nations International Children's Emergency Fund. It was founded in 1946 to address the many health care issues faced by women and children after World War II, and it developed into the best-known social welfare agency in the world. Its original focus on emergency relief has been redefined and expanded to include infrastructure for and delivery of the widest possible range of child health outcomes. At the same time, its outreach has expanded to include families and communities, as so much of children's health is dependent on the health of their society and environment.

In 2018, UNICEF announced the central vision of its 2018–2030 Immunization Roadmap: ensuring that "the right of every woman and every child to immunization is fully realized, with priority given to the most disadvantaged" (UNICEF, 2018). In the previous 30 years, UNICEF had emerged as the operations center for world immunization efforts, providing leadership and advocacy, organizing storage facilities and supply chains, building demand through education and communication, and developing partnerships among communities, local and national governments, and philanthropic agencies. UNICEF's efforts, administered through their field offices, are largely responsible for worldwide gains in vaccination rates. The organization's efforts have also enabled vaccination to become a driver for the provision of other forms of pediatric health care. As parents bring their children to be vaccinated, they can consult with health care professionals about other topics affecting the welfare of their children.

However, as the UNICEF Roadmap notes, significant barriers must be overcome before every woman and every child is fully vaccinated. Paradoxically, one of the barriers to fully equitable vaccine access is the successful implementation of the full range of vaccines that have been developed. Full vaccine coverage is no longer a matter of a few shots given to young children. Instead, full coverage may take 12 to 15 injections ranging in a child's life from a few weeks after birth through adolescence. Even in wealthy, stable communities, it is very hard to convince teenagers to be vaccinated or to get booster shots. It is much harder in communities where parents and teenagers have to work full time, often far away from home.

Logistical difficulties in getting vaccines to people who need them have also increased. Families living in rural or remote areas are dependent on complicated supply networks for all kinds of goods and services; vaccines and syringes are generally fragile to ship and hard to store without existing refrigeration facilities. Families in urban areas, though not geographically distant from vaccines, may still find them inaccessible if the rapid growth of cities has not been matched by a growth in social services. Families in conflict-affected countries, forced into unsafe living conditions and refugee camps, often have to prioritize basics like food, water, and a place to sleep over vaccination schedules. Local epidemics and pandemics like COVID-19 also disrupt other forms of health care, such as vaccinations against other diseases that pose potential threats in the country or region in question.

Rather than insisting on a "one-size-fits-all approach," UNICEF advocates working country by country, region by region, to find the world's most vulnerable women and children and develop vaccination logistics based on their specific needs. The assumption is that children who are not vaccinated are "also not receiving other child survival interventions and are therefore suffering multiple deprivations" (UNICEF, 2018).

Determining why families are not receiving the recommended vaccines—and taking all the steps necessary to make the vaccines accessible—will help minimize the vaccine gap between the global wealthy and the global poor.

FURTHER READING

Africa, World Health Organization (WHO). 2021. "Vaccination boosts Sierra Leone's Ebola prevention." https://www.afro.who.int/news /vaccination-boosts-sierra-leones-ebola-prevention.

Africa, World Health Organization (WHO). 2021. "WHO Supports the Cholera Vaccination Campaign in Zambia's Hot Spot Districts as the Country Accelerates Its Efforts to Eliminate the Deadly Disease." https:// www.afro.who.int/news/who-supports-cholera-vaccination -campaign-zambias-hot-spot-districts-country-accelerates-its.

Burnett, Eleanor, Umesh D Parashar, and Jacqueline Tate. 2020. "Real-World Effectiveness of Rotavirus Vaccines, 2006–19: A Literature Review and Meta-Analysis." *Lancet Global Health* 8: e1195–202. https:// doi.org/10.1016/S2214-109X(20)30262-X.

GAVI, The Vaccine Alliance. n.d. "Rotavirus Vaccine Support." Accessed June 22, 2021. https://www.gavi.org/types-support/vaccine-support/rotavirus.

Pan American Health Organization (PAHO), World Health Organization (WHO). n.d. "Girls in Tarija Receive the HPV Vaccine to Prevent Cervical Cancer." Accessed June 22, 2021. https://www.paho.org/en/stories /girls-tarija-receive-hpv-vaccine-prevent-cervical-cancer.

Pan American Health Organization (PAHO), World Health Organization (WHO). n.d. "Immunization." Accessed June 22, 2021. https://www .paho.org/en/topics/immunization.

United Nations Children's Fund (UNICEF). 2018. *UNICEF Immunization Roadmap 2018–2030.* https://www.unicef.org/sites/default/files/2019-01 /UNICEF_Immunization_Roadmap_2018.pdf.

Vanderslott, Samantha, Bernadeta Dadonaite, and Max Roser. 2019. "Vaccination." *Our World in Data.* https://ourworldindata.org/vaccination.

Western Pacific, World Health Organization (WHO). 2019. "Hong Kong (SAR) Eliminates Rubella." https://www.who.int/westernpacific/news /detail/21-05-2021-hong-kong-sar-(china)-eliminates-rubella.

Western Pacific, World Health Organization (WHO). 2019. "Immunization Gaps Threaten Gains on Measles." https://www.who.int/westernpacific /news/detail/29-03-2019-immunization-gaps-threaten-gains -on-measles.

World Health Organization (WHO). 2020. *Basic Documents.* https://apps .who.int/gb/bd/.

Q21. ARE GOVERNMENTS ESSENTIAL IN MAKING VACCINES EFFECTIVE, SAFE, AND ACCESSIBLE?

Answer: Yes. Governments make vaccines possible in many ways. In vaccine-producing nations, governments often provide much of the funding for research and innovation, whether in government-sponsored laboratories or in the form of grants to university and pharmaceutical company research centers.

In addition, governments throughout the world are the major purchasers of vaccines, which are then distributed to their populations. Vaccines, unlike some other medical products, cannot rely on the free market. They must be produced in specific quantities, and then they must be used within a specific time frame. To ensure that there are enough vaccines every year to immunize all children, protect all essential veterinary workers against rabies, and safeguard all health care professionals again the flu, government agencies work with private companies to guarantee the purchase of a certain number of units. In emergency situations such as the COVID-19 pandemic, governments may prepurchase large numbers of vaccine units to make sure they don't run short.

Governments have an equally important role in regulating vaccines. National regulatory agencies (NRAs) do not get much attention in news media, but they play an essential role in ensuring that vaccines are effective, safe, and accessible. Since the early 2000s, the World Health Organization (WHO) has worked closely with its member nations to set up clear objectives and standards for regulatory agencies. Dr. Mariângela Simão, WHO's assistant director-general for Drug Access, Vaccines, and Pharmaceuticals, noted that health care professionals "expect the products they use to work as described on the box—in fact, to actually be what is described on the box." She emphasized that both health care workers and their patients have "to be able to trust that products . . . actually do what they are meant to do: prevent illness and improve people's health." The best way to ensure that, said Simão, is through good regulatory systems which provide "oversight of health products throughout their life-cycle from the laboratory to the health facility" (WHO, 2019, *Delivering Quality-Assured Medical Products*).

Good regulatory systems are expensive to maintain, and they have tended to flourish in higher-income countries with long histories of public and private support of health care initiatives. Only 50 countries meet the high WHO standards of a "stable, well-functioning, and integrated regulatory system," and a subset of those—including the United States, Canada, and European nations—meet the highest standards of "Regulatory system operating at advanced level of performance and continuous improvement" (WHO, 2019, "Regulatory Systems Strengthening Programme"). Low-income countries, and those in the midst of conflict, face significant challenges to developing stable NRAs, but WHO is committed to working with all member nations to address specific needs.

The Facts: Historically, the regulation of medical products, including vaccines, has been the responsibility of the government of the country where the products were made. In the United States, public outcry over impure vaccines led to the Biologics Control Act of 1902, which established what would become the Food and Drug Administration (FDA). As a result of the Act, companies that manufactured vaccines were required to apply for a license from the government, and as part of the licensing process, government scientists were empowered to inspect laboratory facilities and test products before approval. Over the course of the 20th century, the FDA became a key regulator of new vaccines as they emerged, working closely with the Centers for Disease Control and Prevention (CDC) to set quality-control standards for all aspects of vaccine development, including integrity of the science, purity of ingredients, and safety of clinical trials. Once a new vaccine has been approved, the Advisory Committee on Immunization Practices (ACIP), a committee within the CDC, is responsible for specific recommendations about its safe and effective use.

For most of the century, there was little emphasis on international regulatory standards. Many vaccine-producing countries, as well as some international organizations such as the European Union and the Pan American Health Organization, produced their own sets of regulatory standards. These applied not only to vaccines produced by member nations but also to those that were imported.

In the 1970s, WHO developed the Expanded Programme on Immunization, working with UNICEF and other UN agencies to provide increased access to vaccines in low- and middle-income nations. That meant that it became a major purchaser and distributor in the world vaccine market, which led in turn to WHO developing its own regulations for quality control, including laboratory inspections and testing of vaccines and related products in its own laboratories. As the complexity of vaccine production methods and logistics of distributions increase, so too did the complexity of regulation.

This was more than just a bureaucratic headache. It added to the existing inequity in access to vaccines between high-income and lower and middle-income countries. A 2016 study found that the average time to introduce a new product in low and middle-income countries might be two or three times as much as in a high-income country. The roadblocks include "bottlenecks caused by multistage approval processes, inadequate funding, and different standards and requirements applied by national regulatory authorities" (WHO, 2019, *Delivering Quality-Assured Medical Products*).

WHO therefore turned its attention to creating, in cooperation with member nations, a clear framework for evaluating and strengthening national regulatory agencies. The framework consists of a number of interlocking components: laws passed by government and legal decisions handed down by courts, regulations and guidelines developed by governmental agencies, committees, and oversight boards, and executive decisions by heads of governmental bodies and or national, state, and local governments. In an ideal scenario, all components of this regulatory system would work together, guided by scientific knowledge, to develop best-practices public health policy.

In assessing existing national regulatory systems, WHO relies on nine principles of good regulatory practice:

Legality	Regulatory systems and the decisions that flow from them must have a sound legal basis.
Consistency	Regulatory oversight of medical products should be consistent with existing government policies and legislation and be applied in a consistent and predictable manner.
Independence	Institutions executing regulatory oversight of medical products should be independent.
Impartiality	All regulated parties should be treated equitably, fairly, and free from bias.
Proportionality	Regulation and regulatory decisions should be proportional to risk and the regulator's capacity to implement and enforce.
Flexibility	Regulatory oversight should not be prescriptive but rather allow for flexibility in responding to a changing environment and unforeseen circumstances. Responsiveness in a timely manner to public health emergencies should be built into the regulatory system.
Clarity	Regulatory requirements should be accessible to and understood by users.
Efficiency	Regulatory systems should achieve their goals within the required time and at reasonable effort and cost. International collaboration promotes efficiency by allowing the best use for resources.
Transparency	Regulatory systems should be transparent; requirements and decisions should be made known, and input sought on regulatory proposals. (WHO, 2020)

The goal of these standards is not to penalize countries whose regulatory agencies are not able to meet these principles, but rather to establish benchmarks they can work toward. During the evaluation process, WHO staff meet with personnel from branches of the national regulatory agencies. They identify strengths and weaknesses, working with local staff to develop an institutional development plan to build on the former and address the latter. They emphasize the high priority of good regulatory practices and monitor progress made in achieving regulatory goals.

The benefit of this process became clear in 2018, when the Tanzania Medicines and Medical Devices Authority (TMDA) became the first national regulatory authority in the African region to achieve maturity level three: "Stable, well-functioning, and integrated regulatory system." The TMDA has established and maintained the highest global standards for clinical trials, for regulation of medical products, and for surveillance of medical products once they enter the market. Tanzania medical centers also offer laboratory training to scientists from other African countries, making it much more accessible.

The strength of national regulatory systems is directly linked to vaccination development and distribution, because WHO has a system in place for prequalifying vaccines for use by UNICEF and other UN agencies. That is, manufacturers of specific vaccines can ask in advance that their products be evaluated and cleared for purchase, whenever they might be needed. Since UNICEF purchases millions of vaccine units each year, prequalification is an enormous savings in time and effort. It allows manufacturers to plan in advance for the numbers that might be needed in any given year. It also allows UNICEF to plan for all the logistical hurdles that might need to be overcome, such as access to special storage facilities or transportation networks that can reach across cities, jungles, deserts, and mountains.

In order to submit a vaccine for prequalification, manufactures must be operated in countries whose national regulatory systems have been designated as maturity level three or four. That means that those countries have already put considerable effort into guaranteeing the efficacy and safety of the vaccine. Vaccines and other products are carefully monitored for purity of materials and consistency from batch to batch. The national regulatory authorities keep track of field performance and use high-quality, independent laboratories to assess results. As the countries in which the vaccines are produced already have regulatory authorities that follow all nine principles of good regulatory practice, WHO does not require additional research and evaluation.

Prequalification requires good regulatory practices from vaccine-recipient nations as well. Their national regulatory systems must include two essential features: a set of published requirements for licensing of vaccine products, and capacity for consistent surveillance of vaccine efficacy and safety, once they've been distributed. Prequalification also plays a key role in global Emergency Use Authorizations (EUAs) for vaccines that have been produced quickly to deal with epidemics and pandemics. Vaccines produced under EUAs during the COVID-19 and Ebola outbreaks could be rapidly prequalified and thus made available for global distribution.

In the discussion of vaccines, regulations often seem boring and bureaucratic, taking a backseat to news about scientific discoveries and social and political controversies. But the global regulatory framework established and supported by WHO and member nations is an important reason why vaccines are effective, safe, and reliable. We can trust that doses of vaccines, syringes, and storage facilities are the same whether in New York, Bolivia, Tanzania, Russia, or 190 other countries, because all 194 WHO member nations have agreed to follow the same regulatory standards including legality, consistency, and efficiency. We can trust that surveillance statistics produced in Israel and South Africa and India are relevant to people in Canada, Mexico, and Peru because all countries have agreed to standards of impartiality, clarity, and transparency. The more these national and international regulatory systems work together, the greater the efficacy, safety, and accessibility of the vaccines they supply worldwide.

FURTHER READING

Emamian, Milad, Emily Galik, Allie Gottlieb, Lynn McDonough, and Lila Sevener. 2019. "Regulating Vaccination in the United States." *The Regulatory Review.* https://www.theregreview.org/2019/12/28/saturday-seminar -regulating-vaccination-united-states/.

Khadem Broojerdi, Alireza, Hiiti Baran Sillo, Razieh Ostad Ali Dehaghi, Mike Ward, Mohamed Refaat, and Jane Parry. 2020. "The World Health Organization Global Benchmarking Tool: An Instrument to Strengthen Medical Products Regulation and Promote Universal Health Coverage." *Frontiers in Medicine* 7: 457. https://www.frontiersin.org/articles/10.3389 /fmed.2020.00457/full.

Tanzania Medicines and Medical Devices Authority (TMDA). n.d. "Notable Achievements." Accessed June 25, 2021. https://www.tmda.go.tz/pages /notable-achievements.

World Health Organization (WHO). 2019. *Delivering Quality-Assured Medical Products for All 2019–2023: WHO's Five-Year Plan to Help Build Effective and Efficient Regulatory Systems.* https://apps.who.int/iris/handle /10665/332461.

World Health Organization (WHO). 2021. *Evaluating and Publicly Designating Regulatory Authorities as WHO Listed Authorities.* https://www .who.int/publications/i/item/9789240023444.

World Health Organization (WHO). 2020. "Good Regulatory Practices for Regulatory Oversight of Medical Products. Draft Working Documents

for Comments." https://www.who.int/medicines/areas/quality_safety
/quality_assurance/QAS16_686_rev_3_good_regulatory_practices
_medical_products.pdf.

World Health Organization (WHO). n.d. "Prequalification of Medical
Products (IVDs, Medicines, Vaccines and Immunization Devices, Vec-
tor Control)." Accessed June 24, 2021. https://extranet.who.int/pqweb
/vaccines.

World Health Organization (WHO). n.d. "WHO Regulatory Systems
Strengthening Programme." Accessed June 24, 2021. https://www.who
.int/medicines/technical_briefing/tbs/TBS2019_WHO_RSS_Capacity
_Building_GBT.pdf.

Q22. ARE PHILANTHROPIC ORGANIZATIONS INVOLVED IN MAKING VACCINES SAFE, EFFECTIVE, AND ACCESSIBLE AROUND THE WORLD?

Answer: Yes. Many countries lack funds to either produce or purchase vaccines for their population. This poses dangers not only to citizens vulnerable to vaccine-preventable diseases, but also to the rest of the world, since disease can travel rapidly via global transportation networks. Since the early 2000s, a coalition of public and private funding has worked to ensure that through effective vaccination efforts, local, national, and global communities are protected.

By far the largest, best known, and most effective of these coalitions is GAVI, the Vaccine Alliance. The term GAVI was originally the acronym for Global Alliance for Vaccines and Immunization, the earliest name of the organization. Key stakeholders were the Bill and Melinda Gates Foundation, which contributed $750 million in seed money; the World Health Organization (WHO), which oversaw the Expanded Program in Immunization; the United Nations Children's Fund (UNICEF), which distributes vaccines and associated technologies worldwide; and the World Bank, which provides mechanisms for funding development and healthcare initiatives in lower- to middle-income nations (LMIC). Its official launch was January 31, 2000, at the World Economic Forum in Davos, Switzerland.

GAVI provides funding for large-scale vaccination campaigns to countries the World Bank has defined as lowest-income: as of 2020, those with gross national income (GNI) per capita (by person) of less than $1,630 per year. To put that in perspective, the GNI threshold for a high-income nation is over $12,500. Since 2000, 940 million people have been vaccinated as a direct result of GAVI efforts, bringing the percentage those vaccinated from around 60 percent in 2000 to around 81 percent in 2018. According to impact studies, 13.8 million future deaths have been prevented through GAVI-supported vaccination programs.

GAVI's policies and activities have generated some controversy. The organization has been criticized for being overly influenced by the business and technological practices associated with Bill Gates, the founder of Microsoft. Critics have asserted that in its focus on getting shots into people's arms, GAVI has concentrated on technological improvements rather than looking at ways of addressing basic inequities in health care afflicting poor people in poor countries. It has also not fully addressed the problems of vaccine inequity in middle-income countries. These nations are not eligible to apply for GAVI funding but also not able on their own to provide vaccines for their entire population. GAVI may well have to evolve as it faces continued challenges of ongoing inequities between "vaccine-have" and "vaccine-have-not" nations.

The Facts: The 1990s were a difficult decade for global vaccination programs. WHO's Expanded Programme on Immunization, first launched in 1974, had a global impact through the 1980s, expanding vaccination programs and increasing the numbers of people vaccinated from 5 percent to 50 percent of the population worldwide. But despite massive efforts, progress appeared to stall in the next 10 years.

Part of the reason was scientific innovations in vaccines themselves during the decade. The number of new recommended vaccines increased, and so did the cost of producing and storing them. Governments in high-income countries responded by setting aside a portion of their health care budgets to prepurchasing vaccines, to ensure they would be available for their populations. As major purchasers, year after year, they could negotiate favorable terms with pharmaceutical companies. Governments of lower- to middle-income countries had no such purchasing power. Neither did they have any leverage. As the cost and quantity of recommended vaccines expanded, so did the vaccine gap between have and have-not nations.

Another, related problem had to do with funding for vaccination campaigns. Historically, WHO's vaccination drives had been paid for out of funds provided by member nations, primarily the countries with the highest income. A serious problem with that model was that the amount of funding from each country could fluctuate according to the political or economic climate. But successful vaccination efforts can't afford to fluctuate. Vaccinating all five-year-olds in a country for three years and then skipping the next three cohorts of five-year-olds due to lack of funds is a terrible health care strategy. It does nothing at all for the children who have not been vaccinated, and it may even put the vaccinated children at risk by allowing more dangerous variants to emerge in the nonvaccinated population. To work effectively to reduce the risk of infectious disease, vaccines must be available to everyone, year after year after year.

Inconsistent funding, and the inconsistent purchase pattern that it creates, is also a serious problem on the manufacturing side of vaccine production. Vaccines, like many medical products, arrive at their administration site after a complicated process of production, testing, and storage. Each requires its own set of raw materials, manufacturing facilities, and storage containers. Consistency in demand is therefore a very high priority for pharmaceutical companies, because if they know how many units they need to supply each year, they can correctly gauge the required amount of raw materials and plan for the required manufacturing capacity. If demand fluctuates wildly, they may find themselves with a demand they are unable to meet—or an oversupply they cannot sell. And vaccines cannot be stored indefinitely: each has its own "sell-by" date, after which it will have to be discarded.

GAVI was founded to address these issues. Its revenue stream has three separate components. The first is money provided by donor governments, which make guaranteed pledges to support a high level of funding: over $10 billion from 2000 to 2019. The three largest donors are the United Kingdom, which contributed $2.729 billion from 2000 to 2019; the United States, which contributed $2.469 billion; and Norway, which contributed $1.743 billion. Contributions from Germany, Canada, the Netherlands, and Sweden make up most of the remainder. The second revenue stream comes from private philanthropies, most notably the Bill and Melinda Gates Foundation, which contributed $3.756 billion between 2000 and 2019.

The third funding stream is the most innovative. It is also the one that experts say has made the greatest contribution to GAVI's success. It consists of special "Vaccine Bonds," issued by the World Bank, subject to strict financial regulation, and made available on the international bond markets. They were developed because early efforts made by GAVI continued to be circumscribed by the amount of hard cash available. Donor countries do not deliver all their contributions at once; instead, they may sign an agreement to pay out, for example, a total of $200 million over a period of 20 years. With the guaranteed financial support of these pledges, the World Bank can sell Vaccine Bonds in much the same way that the U.S. government sells savings bonds. The bonds particularly appeal to socially conscious investors. These and other financial instruments have raised over $4 billion between 2006 and 2019.

GAVI has also been able to ensure that the money goes much further by creating a large-volume market for lower-income countries. Prior to 2000, vaccine manufacturers, like other types of manufacturing industries, offered bulk discounts to their high-volume customers, such as government purchasers in high-income countries. The organization's purchasing model tended to lump lower-income countries together as "the rest of the world," with much lower volume and therefore higher prices. By providing UNICEF and its national partners with the resources to make high-volume purchases, GAVI could work with vaccine manufacturers to lower the price per unit. GAVI has also worked to expand the industrial capacity of vaccine manufacturers in lower-income countries, helping to ensure that they meet WHO regulatory standards for prequalification. As a result of both efforts, the unit cost of vaccines has dropped significantly, making them more accessible.

GAVI, like WHO, emphasizes the value of the vaccines for diphtheria, tetanus, and pertussis as the cornerstone of vaccination efforts. It has been a long-standing and successful proponent of the eradication of polio, which is currently found only in small numbers in Afghanistan and Pakistan. The organization has introduced and created stockpiles for chronic diseases such as rotavirus, measles, rubella. It has also helped distribute and stockpile vaccines against diseases prevalent in war-torn areas or those suffering from natural disasters, such as cholera. During the Ebola outbreaks in West Africa in 2014–16, GAVI played a major role in making new vaccines available once WHO had authorized them for emergency use. During the COVID-19 pandemic, GAVI took a leadership role in COVAX, the initiative to ensure that all countries, not just high-income ones, had access to COVID-19 vaccines.

An important component of GAVI's mission is to help countries cycle out of the program, as their economy improves above the GNI threshold. Of the 74 countries that were originally accepted into the GAVI program, 16 have successfully transitioned beyond it. One unintended consequence of GAVI's efforts, however, is that some lower- to middle-income countries that have never been eligible for funding have worse vaccine outcomes than the GAVI-eligible countries below them on the income scale. While vaccine rates among GAVI-eligible countries improve, those with only slightly higher-income levels may be left behind.

GAVI supporters particularly point to its technological innovations. In the 1990s, a very serious problem with vaccination efforts was a severe shortage of syringes. In the absence of other options, health care workers reused syringes, which increased the risk of infections like hepatitis B and hepatitis C. GAVI worked to provide and promote the use of auto-disable syringes, which can only be used once. GAVI also provided technical expertise as well as support for secure, sustainable cold-chain facilities to ensure vaccines could be transported to and stored in remote areas. In Ghana, a very 21st-century success story involved partnering with Zipline and UPS to deliver vaccines via autonomous drones, in order to ensure that the right kinds of vaccines were delivered to the children who needed them in the most efficient way.

These new technologies capture the public's attention, but GAVI's critics have noted that the organization's emphasis on technological achievement may detract from other, more systematic health care reform. GAVI has been criticized for the emphasis placed on polio eradication—not because polio isn't a terrible disease, but because children in low-income nations may suffer much more from malnutrition, lack of clean water, and absence of basic pediatric care. Public health experts have suggested that low-cost, though less exciting, health care interventions might be a better use of international resources. For example, mosquito netting and window screens are effective, low-cost ways of protecting children against insect-borne diseases like malaria and Zika. Wouldn't it make sense to direct international investment to those kinds of solutions, they ask, instead of the millions of dollars needed to develop and produce vaccines?

GAVI's supporters have responded to these criticisms by pointing to the difficulty of using international aid and investment to strengthen entire health care systems, due to the lack of meaningful ways to evaluate success. They also point to data that shows that vaccination infrastructure, once established in a country, can become the basis of meaningful change in primary health care, especially for women and young children. The supply chains, health care workers, medical facilities, and data analysis originally developed for vaccination have been applied to other forms of health care, especially maternal and neonatal care. When parents bring their children for vaccination, or when they come themselves, the visits become opportunities to discover and treat other health issues as well. Philanthropic contributions to vaccination then become the scaffolding upon which more equitable, safe, and effective health care systems can be built.

FURTHER READING

Belluz, Julia. 2015. "The Media Loves the Gates Foundation. These Experts Are More Skeptical." *Vox.* https://www.vox.com/2015/6/10/8760199/gates -foundation-criticism.

GAVI—The Vaccine Alliance. 2019. *Annual Progress Report.* https://www .gavi.org/sites/default/files/programmes-impact/our-impact/apr/Gavi -Progress-Report-2019_1.pdf.

GAVI—The Vaccine Alliance. 2020. *GAVI@20*. https://www.gavi.org
/gavi-at-20.

GAVI—The Vaccine Alliance. 2021. *How We Work Together. Quick Start
Guide for New Members of the Vaccine Alliance*. https://www.gavi.org
/sites/default/files/document/2020/How-we-work-together-feb-2020.pdf.

GAVI—The Vaccine Alliance. 2019. "Immunisation. Strengthening Primary Healthcare for Universal Health Coverage." https://www.gavi.org
/sites/default/files/publications/Immunisation%20-%20a%20platform
%20for%20universal%20health%20coverage.pdf.

Storeng, Katerini. 2014. "The GAVI Alliance and the 'Gates approach' to
Health System Strengthening." *Global Public Health* 9: 865–79. https://
doi.org/10.1080/17441692.2014.940362.

Zerhouni, Elias. 2019. "GAVI, the Vaccine Alliance." *Cell* 179 (1): 13–17.
https://doi.org/10.1016/j.cell.2019.08.026.

Q23. DO ARMED CONFLICTS MAKE IT HARDER FOR PEOPLE TO GET VACCINATED?

Answer: Yes. During the 1960s, a popular anti-war slogan proclaimed,
"War is not healthy for children and other living things." That has been
proven to be true time and time again. Armed conflicts disrupt the lives of
children and many civilian communities in countless ways. Among the
casualties are aspects of life that require peace and a measure of prosperity,
such as schools, medical centers, and childhood and adult vaccinations. In
2018, the Turkish Medical Association took the slogan a step further,
declaring that "war is a man-made public health problem" (Razum et al.,
2019).

During an actual armed conflict, many kinds of nonemergency health
measures take a backseat to simple survival. Civilian families who find
themselves in the midst of fighting take cover immediately, and whomever is
in charge—whether national or local governments or military personnel—
will impose curfews and lockdowns on all nonessential activity. Civilian
health care facilities and personnel may be commandeered for military
purposes. In some cases, civilian populations, including children, may be
targeted. Supply chains for all kinds of medical supplies, including vaccines and cold storage facilities, are likely to be disrupted by fighting.

The indirect effects of armed conflict are even greater. The humanitarian organization Save the Children calculates that children in conflict
zones are three times more likely to die from disease and malnutrition than
bombs and bullets. Two-thirds of the children around the world who have

never received any vaccinations—sometimes called "zero-dose" children— live in areas affected by conflict. During the COVID-19 pandemic, house- holds in the most conflict-ridden areas will be among the last to have access to vaccines.

The United Nations (UN) has issued guidelines on humanitarian aid to war-torn countries, and it includes guidance on vaccination as an essential part of humanitarian care for children and families. Organizations includ- ing the International Federation of Red Cross and Red Crescent Societies (IFRC), Save the Children, and Mercy Corps also provide health care in what are known as fragile, conflict-affected, and vulnerable settings where children are most at risk. All humanitarian organizations work to ensure that, destructive as war may be, it does not completely disrupt the provi- sion of lifesaving vaccines against infectious disease.

The Facts: Since the 19th century, humanitarian organizations have assisted civilians in times of conflict by providing health care and other social services, whether in war-torn communities or refugee camps. As international law evolved over the 19th and 20th centuries, humanitarian activities were protected by legal agreements subscribed to by most coun- tries. The United Nations has brokered many such agreements, including the 1989 Convention on the Rights of the Child, subsequently ratified by 196 countries. This was possible because even nations with very different views on the interpretation of human rights could agree on the value of safeguarding children.

However, in most fragile, conflict-affected, and vulnerable settings, the conflict is not between sovereign nations whose armed forces make a clear distinction between military and civilian personnel. Instead, it is between groups of armed insurgents, which may deliberately target civilian com- munities as a way of spreading terror and maintaining their control over territory. Conflict may also lead to the rise of armed gangs who prey upon the civilian population. And sitting governments have also used armed forces to deliberately target civilians for their ethnic, religious, or cultural identities. During war, atrocities may be committed by all sides.

As a 1996 UN report explained, "Distinctions between combatants and civilians disappear in battles fought from village to village or from street to street. . . . Any and all tactics are employed, from systematic rape, to scorched-earth tactics that destroy crops and poison wells, to ethnic cleansing and genocide." The report continued, "War violates every right of a child—the right to life, the right to be with family and community, the right to health, the right to the development of the personality and the right to be nurtured and protected" (Machel, 1996).

The 1996 report led to the appointment of a Special Representative to the Secretary-General of the UN for children and armed conflict, empowered to gather and verify information and develop action plans for addressing abuses. Many of these abuses are horrific, such as forced recruitment of child soldiers and sexual violence against girls and women.

Though a 2016 UN report found signs of improvement, it also noted increased attacks on health care facilities and personnel. During the Syrian Civil War, for example, which began in 2011, nearly half the hospitals had been destroyed by 2016. Those which remained were filled with injured and dying. Under those circumstances, it was impossible for children to obtain basic health care. In 2010, 80 percent of Syrian children had received all three required doses of diphtheria, tetanus, and pertussis (DTaP) vaccine; by 2018, that number had decreased to 47 percent.

Similar patterns can be seen in other conflict-affected areas. In Iraq, Nigeria, and Yemen, the outbreak of armed conflict is correlated to a significant drop off in the percentage of children who receive basic vaccinations. Reasons for the decline include legitimate fears about civilian safety, destruction of medical facilities, and lack of fuel to maintain cold storage facilities.

Save the Children has outlined the process by which children in conflict-affected areas become most vulnerable to vaccine-preventable disease outbreaks. As conflict breaks out, families try to leave the area, triggering mass population movements. Overcrowding in refugee camps, besieged cities, temporary shelters, and boats leads to diseases associated with poor hygiene, like cholera and rotavirus infections; it also increases transmission rates. Mass movements and temporary housing lead to contaminated food and malnutrition, which makes children more susceptible to vaccine-preventable disease. Measles and rotavirus, which spread more easily in these conditions, also increase susceptibility to disease.

Once conflict breaks out, another common outcome is that health care facilities and personnel are devastated. Routine vaccination, like other kinds of preventative care, is generally stopped altogether as those health care facilities that are not destroyed are turned over to emergency or military needs. Other important vaccination infrastructure, such as equipment depots and cold storage facilities, may be destroyed by conflict or again turned over to other uses. All types of record-keeping that might help track vulnerable and at-risk children are likely to be halted if not completely destroyed.

Governments, which in times of peace play an essential role in funding and providing infrastructure for vaccination programs, become profoundly unstable in times of war. Even if agencies exist to coordinate health care initiatives, staff are unlikely to function effectively in periods of profound insecurity. International organizations may not be allowed access to the region in the midst of fighting. Even if a cease-fire is agreed upon, the greatest need may be for emergency medical and social services. It may take time before the region is stable enough to allow vaccinations to take place.

If outbreaks of vaccine-preventable diseases do occur, they spread rapidly across all vulnerable populations. Through mass movements of populations, the diseases may spread to other, non-combatant regions.

In some cases, vaccination programs are even specifically targeted by militant groups. In Pakistan and Afghanistan, attacks on polio vaccinators derailed eradication efforts in those countries. Al-Shabaab, the militant group that controls much of rural Somalia, has outlawed all vaccines— those against COVID-19 as well as DTaP, measles, and polio. As one observer noted, vaccine distribution in those districts "presents more security challenges than it will help them prevent the disease. Lives are affected at both levels—whether you get killed by them [Al-Shabaab] or by the disease" (Adepoju, 2021).

The COVID-19 pandemic intensified the need for vaccines in conflict-affected areas while also complicating their distribution. The UN called for an end to all global conflicts during the pandemic, so that all nations could focus on fighting the disease. Not surprisingly, that did not happen. To fulfill their mission of ensuring "equitable access to COVID-19 vaccines," therefore, WHO and other humanitarian organizations took as many concrete steps as possible to protect health care workers and allow vaccination to take place. This included reminding governments "that they have a legal and moral responsibility to ensure the health, safety and wellbeing of health workers" (WHO, 2020).

Among the most important security measures was the provision of personal protective equipment, such as gloves and masks, to all health care personnel and any security personnel who accompanied them. Also important was clear communication with humanitarian groups working within the territory, so they could act as mediators with the government or military leadership. Communication was also essential, not just with leaders but also with personnel at every checkpoint and military outpost. Health teams were advised to wear distinctive jackets, badges, T-shirts, and hats to make sure that they could be easily identified as neutral, humanitarian aides. Similar emblems and markings should be visible on cars and temporary medical facilities. There should be an agreed-upon no-weapons policy, and that policy should be exhibited on all cars and facilities. In some cases, it has been possible to negotiate temporary cease-fires to accommodate humanitarian health care, including vaccination.

In conflict-affected regions where there is a clear distinction between military and civilians, military authorities may agree to follow international guidelines for health care. Protecting outbreaks of infectious disease in the civilian population helps to protect their own troops. In northern Nigeria, when ongoing conflict prevented vaccinators from traveling to remote communities, military officers were recruited to drop oral polio vaccines into the mouths of children. In the most remote areas of Mali, vaccinators used to travel by motorcycle, the most effective way to cover the rugged terrain. Due to civil unrest, however, authorities prohibited the use of motorcycles because they are also used by militants. Vaccinators were subsequently forced to travel to unvaccinated families and communities via donkey, horse carts, and dugout canoe. These mechanisms for reaching families can be adapted to providing COVID-19 vaccines to these regions.

In war-torn regions, vaccines can provide emergency care as well as long-term preventive care. Cholera outbreaks are among the most dangerous consequences of warfare. The disease is caused by contaminated food or water. It causes severe diarrhea, and in unhygienic conditions, it can spread like wildfire. Armed conflict often leads to the displacement of large numbers of families, housed in emergency shelters or temporary camps with inadequate water and sanitation facilities. Sometimes combatants even deliberately target water supplies and filtration plants. Yemen reported over one million cases of cholera, and 2500 deaths, between 2016 and 2018. The vaccine against cholera, first invented in the 1980s and approved by the FDA in 2016, has been shown to be highly effective in conflict-affected settings.

Though vaccination in fragile, conflict-affected, and vulnerable areas continues to be precarious, it has the ongoing support of the UN, international law, and humanitarian groups. Advocates hope it can become part of an ongoing, worldwide program to safeguard the health care rights of children and families.

FURTHER READING

Adepoju, Paul. 2021. "The Challenge of Rolling Out Vaccines in African Conflict Zones." *Devex.* https://www.devex.com/news/the-challenge-of -rolling-out-vaccines-in-african-conflict-zones-99932.

Luthi, Eliane. 2019. "Swapping Motorcycles for Donkeys to Deliver Life-Saving Vaccines in Central Mali." *United Nations Children's Fund (UNICEF).* https://www.unicef.org/stories/donkeys-help-deliver-vaccines-mali.

Machel, Graça. 1996. "Impact of Armed Conflict on Children." *United Nations General Assembly.* https://childrenandarmedconflict.un.org/1996/08/1996-graca-machel-report-impact-armed-conflict-children/.

Mercy Corps. 2021. "Countries Facing Highest Levels of Conflict Likely to Be among the Last to Achieve Widespread COVID-19 Vaccination." *Mercy Corps Press Release.* https://www.mercycorps.org/press-room/releases/NPC-Countries-facing-conflict-last-to-receive-vaccine.

Razum, Oliver, Henrique Barros, Robert Buckingham, Mary Codd, Katarzyna Czabanowska, Nino Künzli, Karolina Lyubomirova, Robert Otok, Carlo Signorelli, and John Middleton. 2019. "Is War a Man-made Public Health Problem?" *Lancet* 394 (10209): 1613. https://doi.org/10.1016/S0140-6736(19)31900-2.

Save the Children. 2020. *Not Immune: Children in Conflict.* https://resourcecentre.savethechildren.net/node/18478/pdf/stc01657_immunisation-report_final_oct2020_final-2.pdf?embed=1.

United Nations. General Assembly. 2016. "Report of the Special Representative of the Secretary-General for Children and Armed Conflict." https://www.securitycouncilreport.org/atf/cf/%7B65BFCF9B-6D27-4E9C-8CD3-CF6E4FF96FF9%7D/a_71_205.pdf.

United Nations. Office of the Special Representative of the Secretary-General for Children and Armed Conflict. n.d. *A Mandate to Protect Children Affected by Conflict.* Accessed July 2, 2021. https://childrenandarmedconflict.un.org/wp-content/uploads/2018/04/WEB-EN_Children-and-Armed-Conflict-Office-Brochure-web.pdf.

United Nations Children's Fund (UNICEF). n.d. "Immunisation and Conflict." Accessed July 2, 2021. https://www.unicef.org/immunization/immunization-and-conflict.

United Nations Children's Fund (UNICEF). 2020. "The Lengths to Which Health Workers Go to Reach Every Child with Vaccines." https://www.unicef.org/stories/lengths-which-health-workers-go-reach-every-child-vaccines.

World Health Organization (WHO). 2020. "Keep Health Workers Safe to keep Patients Safe." 17 September 2020. https://www.who.int/news/item/17-09-2020-keep-health-workers-safe-to-keep-patients-safe-who.

World Health Organization (WHO). 2021. "Joint Note on Means to Protect Health Care from Acts of Violence in the COVID-19 Vaccination Rollout in Fragile, Conflict-Affected and Vulnerable Settings." https://www.who.int/publications/m/item/joint-note-on-means-to-protect-health-care-from-acts-of-violence-in-the-covid-19-vaccination-rollout-in-fragile-conflict-affected-and-vulnerable-settings.

Q24. ARE THERE GLOBAL EFFORTS TO PREVENT CRIMES ASSOCIATED WITH VACCINES?

Answer: Yes. Health officials worldwide have long been aware that health care processes are vulnerable to crimes. During times of crisis, such as a pandemic, law enforcement mechanisms and regulatory procedures may be severely disrupted, which in turn means less protection against criminals. Medical supplies, including vaccines, become that much more valuable— and therefore that much more worth stealing and selling on black markets. Huge sums of money pour into government contracts and relief efforts, which leads to increased opportunities for fraud and corruption. Even when there is no health care crisis, the ordinary business of procuring medical supplies, if not closely watched, may open up opportunities for theft, fraud, and corruption.

On October 15, 2020, as the first set of COVID-19 vaccines were completing clinical trials, Secretary-General of the United Nations António Guterres issued a statement against corruption during the pandemic, calling it "criminal, immoral, and the ultimate betrayal of public trust." The virus, he said, had created the kind of worldwide crisis conditions that could lead to crime. "Governments may act in haste without verifying suppliers or determine fair prices," he warned. "Unscrupulous merchants peddle faulty products such as defective ventilators, poorly manufactured tests or counterfeit medicines." He further warned that criminal activity "among those who control supply chains has led to outrageous costs of much-needed goods, skewing the market and denying many people life-saving treatment."

To counteract these bad practices, Guterres advocated for standards of accountability and transparency in government and business practices set out by the United Nations Convention against Corruption, an international, legally binding instrument for combating corruption. Enacted in 2005, it has been signed by 187 states. An important component of the convention is prevention. Countries agree to set standards of accountability and transparency in advance, with effective governmental and civic mechanisms to enforce them. They agree that their law enforcement agencies will cooperate with each other in preventing, investigating, and prosecuting criminals. And they agree to cooperate in recovering assets stolen or obtained by fraud, so that rightful owners and victims of crimes can be compensated.

Secretary-General Guterres called on everyone to assist in the process of combating corruption. "Together," he said, "we must create more robust systems for accountability, transparency and integrity without delay. We must hold leaders to account. Business people must act responsibly. A vibrant civic space and open access to information are essential. And we must protect the rights and recognize the courage of whistle-blowers who expose wrongdoing."

He concluded, "As an age-old plague takes on new forms, let us combat it with new heights of resolve" (Guterres, 2020).

The Facts: To mark International Anti-Corruption Day on December 9, 2020, the United Nations Office on Drugs and Crime (UNODC) issued a policy statement titled "COVID-19 Vaccines and Corruption Risks: Preventing Corruption in the Manufacture, Allocation and Distribution of Vaccines." It drew on lessons learned over the preceding decades, when the World Health Organization (WHO), the United Nations Children's Fund (UNICEF), and other organizations all worked to expand access to vaccines.

An important set of lessons came from the Ebola outbreak in the West African nations of Guinea, Sierra Leone, and Liberia in 2014–16. A total of $124 million had been appropriated by the Red Cross (ICRC) to aid in its relief efforts. However, around $6 million (about 6% of the total) had been lost to a series of crimes ranging from collusion to kickbacks to outright theft. The Red Cross was "outraged" and issued a public statement to insist that it had "zero tolerance for fraud and is committed to full transparency and accountability to our partners and the communities we stand with." The organization's internal accountability measures had turned up "likely collusion" between former Red Cross staff and a bank in Sierra Leone. It had found "over and fake billing by a customs clearance service provider in Guinea." The Red Cross also had uncovered evidence in Liberia of "fraud related to inflated prices of relief items, payroll and payment of volunteer incentives." The statement made it clear that these crimes involved only a small number of merchants and volunteers and that they "must not in any way diminish the tremendous courage and dedication of thousands of volunteers and staff during the Ebola response who worked tirelessly to save countless lives and support families." In subsequent operations, the Red Cross revised its own procedures and worked with international partners to create a stronger bulwark against fraudulent practices (IFRC, 2017).

UNODC's policy paper took a think-tank approach to the risks that corruption and other criminal practices might pose for vaccine development and distribution during the COVID-19 pandemic. That is, they tried to imagine any and all weak points in the process that might provide opportunities for corruption and other criminal practices. Many of these did not, in fact, materialize during COVID-19, in part because public health and governmental officials were aware of weak points and sought to strengthen them.

First are the corruption risks that come from the enormous amounts of money poured into vaccine development. The paper emphasized that, with so much money involved, there had to be procedures in place to ensure that there were no conflicts of interest. People from the pharmaceutical industry who stood to benefit from the contracts should not be able to influence the processes by which those contracts were awarded. An example of this, noted the UNODC, might be "when a high-level officer of a government's COVID-19 vaccine research and development programme, who used to work for a private vaccine company that is bidding for a large contract under the government programme to manufacture a vaccine candidate, participates in a decision making process on that contract."

Another possibility for corruption and fraudulent practices comes from vulnerabilities in the distribution system for vaccines. Vaccines might be "stolen from the public supply chain during the transportation process and diverted to the black market or kept for personal use." Even when they reach their intended health care facility, vaccine supplies may not be safe, "if there are no reliable oversight measures in place. Public health facility staff may also steal vaccines for resale in the black market or in their own private practices." Of course, that is most likely to happen "when supplies are limited, and demand is high, as is the case during a pandemic."

One of the greatest risks of corruption, according to UNODC data, comes from vaccine procurement, the processes involved in ordering and receiving vaccine shipments. At the beginning of the process, "corruption risks include inaccurately estimating the demand for a particular product or service," circumventing standard bidding procedures, and deliberately tailoring official documents "to favour a particular bidder." During the actual bidding, "there is the risk of government officials receiving bribes or kickbacks from suppliers, as well as the risk of collusion and market division between bidders themselves." At the end of the process, "corruption risks include false invoicing, changing contract agreements, and the failure to deliver procured vaccines" (UNODC, "COVID-19 Vaccines and Corruption Risks").

Another risk is the possibility of substandard or outright fake vaccines being marketed, especially by organized criminal groups. During the COVID-19 pandemic, international law enforcement agencies monitored the activities of these groups, including the Mafia, yakuza, and Mexican cartels. They noted an upturn in smuggling of fake and substandard medical products and pharmaceutical supplies, especially as international lockdowns impeded the usual criminal activities of these groups, such as drugs and arms smuggling.

Yet another risk comes from nepotism and favoritism in allocation of available vaccines. Government officials have been known to use their influence to allocate or sequester scarce medical supplies for their own friends and supporters, either to protect themselves from disease or as a way of obtaining political or other favors.

As the COVID-19 vaccine rollout progressed, it was clear that some of these forms of corruption had been adequately guarded against. The vaccines had been developed with careful attention to accountability and transparency, so that although there were policy questions, there were no serious accusations of corrupt practices. Shipment and distribution were also carefully guarded, so that organized crime groups were generally not successful in infiltrating the legitimate vaccine market.

However, many other kinds of criminal behavior did flourish during the pandemic. In countries where populations do not have easy access to accurate health care information, vaccination efforts were bedeviled by all kinds of fraud. These included online and door-to-door scams to obtain personal information while purporting to set up vaccine appointments. Later scammers charged huge fees to set up appointments, claiming to have privileged access. As vaccines became available to some groups, health care workers, both real and fraudulent, charged even more enormous fees to administer what often turned out to be fake vaccines.

In India, as government-authorized vaccinations increased, so did fraudulent activity involving fake vaccines. In July 2021, doctors and other staff at one medical facility were arrested for allegedly injecting thousands of patients with saline solution—water and salt—instead of the COVID-19 vaccine. The health care facility issued false vaccination certificates as well. Patients became suspicious when they compared their own vaccination certificates with the images of real government-authorized versions online. They also wondered why no one who had been vaccinated in this facility experienced side effects. Law enforcement officials believe more than 2,600 people were taken in by the fraud. They were charged between $7 and $10 for the shots, which should have been administered at no charge. Authorities stated that they confiscated $20,000 from the suspects.

Brazil, another country hit hard by the pandemic, has also faced accusations of corruption. In April 2020, tribal leaders of the Yanomami people, in the Amazon region, complained to the government officials that some health workers were trading vaccines for illegally mined gold. A much more widespread scandal erupted in June, when a government commission appointed to review procurement for COVID-19 vaccines became suspicious about a $320 million purchase for 20 million doses of the Covaxin vaccine, manufactured by the India company Bharat Biotech.

The case followed the pattern of other vaccine procurement corruption, as set out by the UNODC policy paper. The contract had been issued quickly, without transparency or explanation. The cost was higher than had been negotiated by other governments. The Covaxin vaccine was still in clinical trials and had not yet been authorized for emergency use. And this quick, costly decision had been made even though Pfizer-BioNTech had been offering its fully authorized vaccine for months and had been refused. These accusations of corruption were politically costly for Brazil's president, Jair Bolsonaro. They showed, however, the value of having policies in place to prevent fraud, in that the alleged corruption was uncovered by the governmental commission empowered to investigate contracts.

As lessons learned during the Ebola outbreak helped strengthen anticorruption measures in place during the COVID-19 pandemic, so it is likely that lessons learned from COVID-19 will strengthen future anticorruption efforts. These may include developing laws and policies to minimize opportunities for special interests, fraud, and kickbacks; improving mechanisms for regulating weak links in the processes by which vaccines are purchased and distributed; and protecting individuals and communities who are most at risk of being targeted for fraud and other kinds of criminal activity.

FURTHER READING

Guterres, António. 2020. "Corruption Is the ultimate betrayal of public trust." *United Nations Covid-19 Response.* https://www.un.org/en/corona virus/statement-corruption-context-covid-19.

International Federation of Red Cross and Red Crescent Societies (IFRC). 2017. "IFRC Statement on Fraud in Ebola Operations." https://media .ifrc.org/ifrc/ifrc-statement-fraud-ebola-operations/.

Kumer, Harry. 2021. "Indian Police Investigate Whether Scammers Gave Thousands of Shots of Salt Water instead of Vaccine." *New York Times.* https://www.nytimes.com/2021/07/04/world/asia/india-covid-vaccine -scam.html.

Londoño, Ernesto, and Flávia Milhorance. 2021. "Brazil Vaccine Scandal Imperils Bolsonaro as Protests Spread." *New York Times.* https://www .nytimes.com/2021/07/03/world/americas/brazil-bolsonaro-vaccine -scandal.html.

Paraguassu, Lisandra, and Ricardo Brito. 2021. "Brazil Investigates Reports of Vaccines Being Exchanged for Illegal Gold." *Reuters.* https://www.reuters.com /world/brazil-investigates-reports-vaccines-being-exchanged-illegal -gold-2021-04-14/.

Sullivan, Shane. 2021. "Latin America Sees Rise in Vaccine-related Crimes." *InSight Crime.* https://insightcrime.org/news/vaccine-arrivals -deliver-new-scams-latin-america/.

United Nations Office on Drugs and Crime (UNODC). n.d. "Covid-19 Vaccines and Corruption Risks: Preventing Corruption in the Manufacture, Allocation and Distribution of Vaccines." Accessed July 8, 2021. https://www.unodc.org/documents/corruption/COVID-19/Policy _paper_on_COVID-19_vaccines_and_corruption_risks.pdf.

United Nations Office on Drugs and Crime (UNODC). n.d. "The Impact of COVID-19 on Organized Crime." Accessed July 8, 2021. https://www .unodc.org/documents/data-and-analysis/covid/RB_COVID_organized _crime_july13_web.pdf.

Q25. ARE THERE ONGOING EFFORTS TO PROMOTE VACCINE AWARENESS?

Answer: Yes. Public health campaigns to promote awareness of the benefits of vaccination have been around since the introduction of the smallpox vaccine in the early 19th century. They may be sponsored by local, national, and international public health organizations. Although some may be created by health care professionals, it is more common nowadays for health organizations to partner with or hire communications professionals. These may include writers and artists, public relations and communication specialists, and anthropologists and medical ethicists. By growing and sustaining public trust in vaccines, they play an important role in local, national, and global immunization efforts.

These public awareness campaigns have historically taken two separate approaches, one intended for health care professionals and the other for patients. Public health campaigns for health care professionals are found in scientific journals and outreach programs developed by professional organizations like the American Medical Association and the American Nurses Association. Awareness campaigns can also be incorporated into the ongoing medical education required for many types of professionals. Nowadays, ongoing education is often delivered in the form of webinars with online Question and Answer (Q and A) sessions, as well as tests and other assessments.

Vaccine awareness campaigns for the general public have historically taken advantage of the popular media outlets of the day. During the early 20th century, public health officials wrote articles and inserted public safety announcements in newspapers. They partnered with businesses to produce pamphlets and insert ads in popular magazines read by parents and children. From the 1930s through the 1950s, vaccination awareness campaigns made use of the power of radio to reach homes across the United States and even around the world. During the second half of the century, television took over as the medium of choice for all kinds of public health campaigns. By early in the 21st century, however, the internet and social media had taken over as the main platforms for promoting vaccine awareness. Vaccine information intended for public benefit can now be found freely available on a wide range of websites, with downloads and links to top social media sites such as Facebook, Instagram, Twitter, and YouTube.

During the COVID-19 pandemic, the World Health Organization (WHO) promoted its vaccine awareness campaign with the slogan "Vaccines Bring Us Closer" and the Twitter hashtags #VaccinesWork and #GetVax. The Ministry of Information and Broadcasting in India used #We4Vaccine. The Australian Government Department of Health kept its messaging simple: #COVID19Vaccine and a graphic with their slogan "COVID-19 VacciNA-TION." As the vaccine rollout progressed, newly vaccinated people responded with their own social media posts and hashtags, declaring #IGotTheShot and #VaccinesSaveLives.

The Facts: The media campaign to build public awareness for the polio vaccine set the standard for many of the public health campaigns that followed. During the first half of the 20th century, polio was one of the most feared diseases in the United States. Polio struck approximately 35,000 Americans every year, with once-healthy children accounting for a large number of the overall cases. The disease left many victims crippled or weakened for life. It appeared to strike out of nowhere, especially in the summer months, when children played and swam together in neighborhoods and in summer camps. During such outbreaks, public health officials closed pools and playgrounds, and many communities imposed travel restrictions.

In 1921, a promising young lawyer and aspiring politician named Franklin Delano Roosevelt was vacationing on his yacht in Canada. When he lost his balance and fell into the water, he scrambled back on board immediately with no apparent ill effects. Three days later, however, he was no longer able to stand, and his doctors diagnosed polio. Despite daily efforts to regain his ability to walk, he spent most of the rest of his life in a wheelchair. This setback did not stop his political career, however. Roosevelt went on to serve as governor of New York State from 1928 to 1932 and then as president of the United States from 1932 to 1945, where he guided the country through both the Depression and World War II.

When the newly formed Society for Infantile Paralysis was formed in 1938, Roosevelt was an obvious choice to serve as sponsor. He announced its founding in a speech broadcast across the country via radio, a new form of that which the president had successfully harnessed for public outreach. He described the many small contributions of dimes and quarters he had received in 40,000 letters from children who wanted to see other children get well. The March of Dimes, as the Society for Infantile Paralysis came to be known, took up that image in its fundraising. The organization used radio and print advertising campaigns to urge children to collect dimes for research to find a polio vaccine and cure.

The Food and Drug Administration (FDA) approved the first polio vaccine administered by injection in 1955. Eight years later, the FDA approved a vaccine that could be administered orally, on a sugar cube. The March of Dimes adapted its fundraising campaigns toward education, crafting messages to convince mothers to vaccinate their children. The March of Dimes recruited an army of mothers—many of whom had donated their dimes as children—to go door to door in their neighborhoods, promoting the value of the polio vaccine. The organization took out ads in newspapers, magazines, and on radio. It also recruited television hosts and celebrities to promote vaccination with special events. For example, the popular music star Elvis Presley appeared on the Ed Sullivan Show with a little girl who had contracted polio. Presley then got his own polio vaccination shot while on camera. By the 1960s, the number of polio cases in the United States had fallen to approximately 100 per year, and by the 1970s, it fell to 10 cases annually. In 1979, polio was declared eliminated in the United States.

Rather than focusing on specific diseases, the Centers for Disease Control and Prevention (CDC) currently sponsor events to promote public awareness of vaccines. These include National Infant Immunization Week (NIIW) in April, National Immunization Awareness Month (NIAM) every August, and National Influenza Vaccination Week (NIVW), held in early December at the start of flu season.

At the start of the 21st century, the CDC still focused on the traditional media outlets of newspapers, magazines, radio, and television. The media toolkit provided for the 2011 Influenza Awareness Campaign gave detailed information for promoting the campaign through "print and Internet ads, matte articles, TV and radio public services announcements, personal testimony videos featuring parents who have been greatly affected by influenza, radio interviews," sound bites, "special events, and collaboration with partners" (CDC, 2011).

The 23-page toolkit provided detailed information on how to develop a public awareness campaign. The first step was to ensure that the CDC's key messages—the main points of the campaign—were consistent throughout the media materials. The messages for influenza emphasized the seriousness of the disease, the vulnerability of certain populations, such as older people and young children, the need to protect families, and the numbers of people—hundreds of millions—who had safely received the seasonal flu vaccines. The second step was to create press materials, many of which were available in standard formats from the CDC. These included one-page press releases, public service announcements (PSAs) for local radio and television stations, letters to the editor, and news conferences and other special events. Each has its own format. Each had its own format. For example, the CDC provided PSAs of 15, 30, and 60 seconds in length, with titles such as "Why Flu Vaccination Matters: Personal Stories of Families Affected by Flu," "I Never Get the Flu," and "Flu Ends with U," available in English and Spanish.

The next steps dove into the logistics of media campaigns. The third step, "Preparing for Outreach," urged partners to develop spreadsheets of media contacts arranged by type, such as newspaper or television. It also encouraged them to establish and maintain contacts with other outreach organizations such as "Medical center or clinic newsletters, Supermarket or pharmacy news handouts, Faith-based organization publications . . . Community newsletters, Public health journals, Business journals," school newsletters and newsletters from parent-teacher associations, and bilingual publications. Step four gave instructions on "Training Your Spokespeople," with appendixes to provide how-to information on practicing public speaking skills. Step five was "Pitching the Media," including more tips and tricks on how to interest local media in printing and broadcasting press releases and PSAs about influenza vaccines (CDC, 2011).

Detailed as this was, by 2010 the emphasis on print, radio, and television was no longer cutting edge. By the 2015 flu season, the CDC's two-page information sheet for partners focused primarily on digital media, using an app called Thunderclap, a crowd-speaking program that made it easy for grassroots organizers to promote a message and have social media followers amplify it. National influenza awareness partners were assumed to have a Twitter account, which they could connect to Thunderclap. All messages sent from the CDC Thunderclap account would be automatically shared by its Twitter followers. The CDC hosted a Twitter chat and distributed "NIVW-specific tweets" to its partners, together with the hashtag #NIVW2015. CDC updates were shared with partners via "emails, online reports, and a telebriefing." Finally, the CDC purchased "a Google keyword search and display . . . to raise awareness that everyone 6 months of age and older should get vaccinated. Keyword searches related to flu will trigger

CDC flu vaccination messages to be featured at the top of Google searches. CDC messages will link consumers to the CDC flu website" (CDC, 2015).

By 2021, Thunderclap had been discontinued, and the CDC had streamlined and updated its entire website to accommodate modern internet and social media practices. Information on NIAM was available as downloads from its dedicated CDC webpage, with a separate, downloadable "Toolkit for Reaching Healthcare Professionals" and "Toolkit for Reaching Parent and Patients." Newsletter templates, information items, and web- and social media–friendly graphics were also available for download. NIVW had its own web page and dedicated digital toolkit, with a special @CDC-Flu Twitter handle and many social media hashtags for Facebook, Instagram, and LinkedIn: #FightFlu, #SleeveUp, #MaskUp, #LatherUp. Other tools for the modern public awareness campaign include infographics, GIFs, videos, and podcasts, as well as the now tried-and-true radio PSAs, optimized for local communities and vulnerable populations.

"With all eyes on vaccines," in April 2021, WHO promoted their annual vaccine awareness program, World Immunization Week, as "an unprecedented opportunity to build public trust in the value of all vaccines and help build long-term support for immunization" (WHO, 2021). Their campaign, with the theme Vaccines Bring Us Closer, included a dedicated webpage with links to About the campaign, World champions, and Campaign materials. The key messages connected to what the world had experienced, and in many places was still experiencing, during the COVID-19 pandemic. The first was "Vaccines bring us closer to doing what we love with those we love," a message that resonated with many after over a year of enforced lockdowns and restrictions on gatherings and travel. The second was "Vaccines bring us closer to a world where no one suffers or dies from a vaccine-preventable disease." This messaging moved beyond COVID-19 to serve as a reminder that many children and adults, through lack of access, were not receiving recommended vaccinations. The third area of emphasis was to convey the message that "Vaccines bring us closer to a healthier, more prosperous world." Vaccine-preventable diseases come with a measurable cost, not only in terms of illness and death, but also because a healthy population is a more productive population (WHO, 2021).

WHO's 2021 World Immunization Week was digitally savvy, using Twitter and Instagram hashtags, graphics and GIFs, and links to YouTube videos. Each reiterated the key message: that vaccines bring us closer to the end of the COVID-19 pandemic, to each other, and to the end of mortality, morbidity, and economic loss caused by vaccine-preventable diseases.

FURTHER READING

Bolton, Felicia. 2021. "COVID-19 Vaccine Hashtags Connect People through Social Media." *NewsNation*. https://www.newsnationnow.com /us-news/midwest/covid-19-vaccine-hashtags-connect-people-through -social-media/.

Centers for Disease Control and Prevention (CDC). 2011. *CDC Influenza Awareness Campaign Media Relations Toolkit*. https://www.cdc.gov/flu /pdf/nivw/NIVW_Media_Toolkit_112011.pdf.

Centers for Disease Control and Prevention (CDC). 2015. *CDC Update: 2015–2016 Flu Season. National Influenza Vaccination Week 2015*. https:// www.cdc.gov/flu/pdf/nivw/nivw-activities-12-01-2015.pdf.

Centers for Disease Control and Prevention (CDC). 2020. "National Influenza Vaccination Week." https://www.cdc.gov/flu/resource-center/nivw /index.htm.

Funakoshi, Minami, and Ally J. Levine. 2021. "Speed and Trust. Keys to an Effective Vaccination Program." *Reuters*. https://graphics.reuters.com /HEALTH-CORONAVIRUS/VACCINE-ROLLOUT/rlgvdegqqpo/.

Oshinsky, David. 2006. *Polio: An American Story*. New York: Oxford University Press.

World Health Organization (WHO). 2021. "World Immunization Week 2021." https://www.who.int/campaigns/world-immunization-week/2021.

4

Vaccination Controversies

INTRODUCTION

This section explores aspects of vaccines and vaccination programs that have led to public controversy. What is vaccine misinformation, and can anything be done to counteract it? What are conspiracy theories, and why do they flourish in times of crisis? Can legitimate public concerns about vaccine safety be weaponized by bad actors who make fraudulent claims? Can vaccines be made compulsory? Can they be required in health care settings? Is parental consent required for vaccination of children? What recourse do people have if they believe they or their children have suffered adverse effects from vaccines?

In the course of history, vaccines have sometimes been controversial, but the type of controversy has changed based on prevailing political, social, and scientific issues of the era. During the 18th century, when techniques of smallpox inoculation were just beginning to be understood, the process meant that inoculated patients were still contagious for several weeks. Some communities were therefore opposed to the practice, believing that it increased the risk of contagion for everyone else. For example, the Commonwealth of Virginia discouraged the practice when Thomas Jefferson was a boy, so as a young man he traveled to Pennsylvania, where it was legal, in order to be inoculated.

In the early 19th century, Edward Jenner developed a new vaccination procedure for smallpox that ensured that the recipient was not contagious and could not spread the disease. That became the standard for new types of vaccines over the next 200 years. Nowadays, few communities object to the availability of vaccines in and of themselves. Nor do they object to individual adults becoming vaccinated if they choose to do so. In many circumstances, vaccination is treated as a form of health care, with the decision about whether to vaccinate or not left up to the individual.

In the modern world, the main controversies about vaccines have to do with vaccination programs—particularly about whether they should be made mandatory or not, and if so, under what circumstances. Many countries and regions require a set of childhood vaccinations in order for children to attend public, and some private, schools and universities. Educational institutions, health care facilities, and employers of all kinds may establish their own rules requiring vaccination for their employees and, in many cases, for their patrons and clients. National, regional, and local governments may set their own requirements for all institutions that are regulated by public health laws and codes. Individuals and organizations have challenged many of these public health requirements, contending that they infringe on individual freedoms.

In the United States, vaccination requirements have been upheld in court for more than 100 years, and they have an overall high public approval rating, especially during the COVID-19 pandemic. The same laws that support those requirements also protect the right of individuals to determine their own health care, so that those who choose not to be vaccinated for medical or religious reasons can apply for exemptions from vaccination requirements. Like many legal and political compromises, this has been criticized by people from both sides. There are some who would like to see no exemptions of any sort from vaccination requirements, and others who would like to see no vaccination requirements at all.

The COVID-19 pandemic brought a new intensity to this and other debates. This debate was complicated, however, with the prevalence of misinformation, disinformation, and conspiracy theories in news and social media—much of it seemingly motivated by political considerations.

Misinformation is inaccurate, misleading, or false news or information that is disseminated in the mistaken belief that it is accurate. People and outlets that spread misinformation do not realize that the information is wrong, false, or incomplete.

Disinformation is the purposeful, deliberate spread of false or misleading information—or outright lies—by bad actors, usually for some ulterior purpose or in service to a personal agenda. During the COVID-19 pandemic, this "infodemic" of misinformation and disinformation caused so much damage to efforts to combat the virus that the U.S. Surgeon General issued warnings about it, and major social media outlets took steps to reduce or eliminate it from their platforms.

Other controversies that had been debated for some time reemerged in the course of the COVID-19 pandemic. At what age should individuals be allowed to make their own decisions about vaccination? Not only does the law vary from country to country and from region to region within countries, but also there are differences of opinion between what laws may say and what health care personnel think is in the best interest of their patients. Should doctors dismiss from their practices those families in which parents refuse to vaccinate their children? And if they do, does that make it more or less likely that parents will change their minds? In many vaccine-producing countries, there are specific "vaccine courts" in place to address the complaints of those who believe the vaccines caused adverse effects. In most cases they were set up as a political compromise: patients can be reasonably certain of compensation for a specific set of injuries, but they agree not to sue pharmaceutical companies in civil court. Does this system work as well as its proponents intended? Or is more effort needed to protect the rights of all consumers?

As new types of vaccines emerge to face new medical challenges, it is likely that new controversies will emerge as well.

Q26. ARE VACCINE MISINFORMATION AND DISINFORMATION DANGEROUS?

Answer: Yes. Misinformation is something that pretends to be information—that is, actual facts about a topic—but is not based on any scientific evidence or experience. It tends to flourish during periods of uncertainty, such as during fast-moving epidemics and pandemics, when actual scientific evidence may be limited, and where legitimate scientists may not be able to answer every question until they have conducted the requisite careful research.

Under those circumstances, it is a well-known feature of social behavior that people will try to construct some sort of explanation that covers the many gaps in their knowledge. Even when spread by word of mouth, these kinds of local, socially based explanations can be dangerous. They have been linked to hate speech and crimes for hundreds of years. They can become even more dangerous when amplified and manipulated by media. The best-known media manipulation campaigns are often political in nature, such as the campaigns by Russian secret service operatives to affect elections in the United States, Sweden, and Taiwan. But they can have a medical impact as well. The 1985 media manipulation campaign Operation Denver, carried out by the Russian and East German secret services, was designed to convince South Africans that AIDS and the human immunodeficiency virus (HIV) that caused it had been produced in laboratories in the United States. It contributed to the delay in effective response to the disease in that country and to the deaths of 300,000 people (Kramer, 2020).

Nowadays, an ever-increasing number of people around their world get their information from the internet, and that has led to a huge upswing in media manipulation on many topics, vaccines included. The World Health Organization (WHO) has labeled widespread circulation of false information about COVID-19 and the vaccines developed to fight the pandemic an "infodemic," defined as "too much information, including false or misleading information, in digital and physical environments during a disease outbreak." WHO warned that these falsehoods and misunderstandings lead to "confusion and risk-taking behaviours that can harm health. It also leads to mistrust in health authorities and undermines the public health response." By intensifying mistrust and confusion at a time of crisis, "An infodemic can intensify or lengthen outbreaks when people are unsure about what they need to do to protect their health and the health of people around them" (WHO, "Infodemic").

In a number of vaccination programs worldwide, online misinformation and disinformation have been blamed for disruptions and delays in making vaccines available to vulnerable children. During the COVID-19 pandemic, misinformation campaigns on social media have been linked to low rates of vaccination, which in turn contributed to sharp increases in cases, hospitalizations, and death.

The Facts: Misinformation has been defined as "false information that's shared by people who don't realise it is false and don't mean any harm." It can still be dangerous, though, because it has the power to "dilute, distract, [and] distort" actual, verifiable facts. Disinformation is "deliberately engineered and disseminated false information with malicious intent or to serve agendas." These agendas can be "personal, political, or economic" in nature (UNICEF, 2020).

Many forms of media, such as newspapers, advertising, radio, and television, went through periods in their early history when they spread misinformation or disinformation. In print media, this took the form of sensational, untrue stories, written and published to sell more newspapers or magazines and thus gain more advertisers and advertising revenue. It also took the form of false advertising, in which exaggerated or outright false claims were made for certain products. Newspapers and magazines also trafficked in the publication of false medical information, including articles written by alleged "medical experts" attacking scientific research and knowledge in order to sell their home remedies.

Over time, a combination of laws, government regulations, and professional ethics developed to ensure accountability and punishment for any publishing or broadcasting medium that knowingly spreads inaccurate information in order to sell products. The Federal Trade Commission (FTC) prohibits unfair or deceptive advertising on any medium. The Food and Drug Administration (FDA) has regulations prohibiting deceptive or incomplete advertising about medical products. Moreover, publishing or broadcasting downright inaccurate information is a violation of codes of professional conduct and might well lead to lawsuits, especially if it leads to harm for those who read, listen, or watch. Although these regulations and codes of conduct have not completely eliminated medical misinformation in print media, radio, and television, they have limited it.

The internet is a different matter. Laws and government regulations penalizing false advertising and other fraudulent and criminal activities still apply. However, the major platforms from which people derive information, including Facebook, Twitter, Instagram, and YouTube, cannot be held legally accountable for whatever people post, any more than telecommunications companies can be held accountable for what people say on the phone.

Many people assert that the internet should be as free and unregulated as possible, as though it were a giant corkboard open to everyone's opinions. But what if some people, wealthier or more influential than others, were able to take over more and more of the corkboard? What if they could coordinate their messages and weaponize them, to support those ideas they approved of and attack those they disliked? What if they could manipulate posts, tweets, images, and videos to drive more traffic to their websites and raise more money?

During the past 20 years, there have been many examples of this kind of behavior. Bad actors purvey disinformation about medical issues to fundraise for political or social causes, to link to websites that sell health care products, or simply to raise their own profiles as internet influencers. Medical misinformation and disinformation can be especially useful for those who wish to weaponize media attention, because people are more likely to click on posts that cause worry and alarm than those that are calm and happy.

The United Nations Children's Fund (UNICEF) has documented misinformation and disinformation campaigns that did real, measurable harm to vaccination initiatives designed to protect vulnerable children. In 2018, for example, Pakistan was on track to completely eradicate polio. In 2019, however, Pakistan's polio vaccination efforts were badly damaged by a disinformation campaign whose architects posted videos of unconscious boys in hospitals, together with a voice-over declaring that the boys had gotten sick as a result of the polio vaccine. There was no evidence for this claim, but many Pakistani communities have a long history of vaccine hesitancy, and the videos were taken to be true. Within 24 hours, the videos had garnered 24,000 interactions, and they were amplified by Facebook and WhatsApp. By the end of the week, 45,000 children had been taken to hospitals by their worried parents, fearful that they had been injured by the polio vaccine. A mob of 500 people even attacked a clinic in Peshawar, leading to the deaths of a health care worker and two police officers. Though public health officials tried to stop the rumors with their own announcements, their posts were attacked as a cover-up and otherwise distorted by supporters of the disinformation campaign.

Public health officials sent their most trusted community vaccinators to the districts most affected by the disinformation. These vaccinators worked with community leaders and with families to show that the videos and associated rumors were untrue, and to regain trust in polio vaccines. However, the impact of the videos, followed closely by the COVID-19 pandemic, disrupted Pakistan's polio vaccination program. Unfortunately, as of 2021, Pakistan and Afghanistan persist as the last two countries where polio is endemic.

Another case highlights both the dangers of misinformation, especially when presented in visual form, and how to counteract it. In the early 2010s, the introduction of the human papillomavirus (HPV) vaccine for girls in school settings encountered roadblocks in Denmark and Ireland. In both countries, the vaccine was successfully introduced, but vaccine hesitancy shot up when local television networks aired a video claiming that the vaccine was associated with adverse effects. The airing of the video is considered to be a case of disseminating misinformation rather than disinformation, as the stations thought they were providing a balanced perspective on arguments for and against the vaccine. However, they did not properly investigate their sources for trustworthiness or verifiability, so they ended up airing rumors and conjecture rather than fact. After the airing of this misinformation, the rate of HPV vaccines declined by as much as 50 percent, with many more parents expressing fears of side effects of the vaccine.

Public health authorities took an active role in investigating the rumors, putting into place health care teams that worked directly with schools and parents to alleviate fears of the vaccine. They also stressed the value of the vaccine in preventing cervical cancer. The intervention was successful, and the vaccination rate returned to its previous level.

When UNICEF set out to introduce the HPV vaccine into its clinics in Malawi in 2018, the organization already had considerable experience of the ways in which rumors could derail a vaccination program. Before vaccinating a single child, UNICEF officials established a vaccine crisis communication plan designed to identify, contain, and limit the negative effects of rumors and misperceptions before they spread. They educated all their health service personnel, as well as teachers, media professionals, and community leaders, about rumors and how they spread. They set up a system whereby rumors and misinformation could be rapidly reported, and staff members in the field could be notified about the best way to address any misunderstandings and inaccurate information. Key to the program was active social listening, keeping track of what was trending on social media and developing a rapid response. Community health service workers organized a range of communication activities, including plays and community meetings, to educate the public about the value of HPV for girls' health and well-being. By 2021, 65 percent of the girls in previously hesitant districts had received the vaccine.

During the COVID-19 pandemic, there was tremendous public outcry against the range and persistence of medical misinformation and disinformation online. Digital analysis of anti-vaccine posts found that a substantial number of posts came from media manipulators, deploying an unknown number of paid and volunteer digital hacks and bots to amplify their message. Their posts and tweets link back to sales and fundraising websites and, in some cases, have led to investigations of fraud.

Although the major internet platforms had set up rules to prevent inaccurate or misleading posts, they had seldom been enforced. From 2020 on, repeated requests from their users and employees, as well as the threat of more government regulation, led Twitter, Facebook, Instagram, and YouTube to finally crack down on repeat misinformation offenders. These ranged from flagging posts, tweets, images, and videos that conveyed inaccurate medical information about COVID-19 and vaccination to removing accounts of those who continued to post misleading or incorrect information. By August 2021, Facebook's vice president of content policy, Monica Bickert, stated they had removed over 20 million pieces of content, and more than 3,000 accounts, for breaking their rules about posting COVID-19 misinformation "that could contribute to a risk of someone spreading or contracting the virus" (Bickert, 2021).

Guy Rosen, Facebook's vice president for Integrity, also pointed out that the platform had been a powerful tool for vaccine advocates. "More than

2 billion people have viewed authoritative information about COVID-19 and vaccines on Facebook," he noted. "This includes more than 3.3 million Americans using our vaccine finder tool to find out where to get a COVID-19 vaccine and make an appointment to do so." In addition, "more than 50% of people in the U.S. on Facebook have already seen someone use the COVID-19 vaccine profile frames, which we developed in collaboration with the U.S. Department of Health and Human Services and the CDC. From what we have seen, when people see a friend share they have been vaccinated, it increases their perceptions that vaccines are safe" (Rosen, 2021).

These findings provide support for the idea that if 21st-century social media can evolve into a position of assuming greater social responsibility for the content on their platforms, it can also evolve from being part of the problem of vaccine misinformation to part of the solution.

FURTHER READING

Bickert, Monica. 2021. "How We're Taking Action against Vaccine Misinformation Superspreaders." Facebook. https://about.fb.com/news/2021/08/taking-action-against-vaccine-misinformation-superspreaders/.

Center for Countering Digital Hate. 2020. *The Disinformation Dozen. Why Platforms Must Act on Twelve Leading Anti-Vaxxers.* https://www.counterhate.com/disinformationdozen.

Donovan, Joan, Brian Friedberg, Gabrielle Lim, Nicole Leaver, Jennifer Nilsen, and Emily Dreyfuss. 2021. *The Media Manipulation Case Book.* Harvard Kennedy School, Shorenstein Center on Media, Politics, and Public Policy. https://mediamanipulation.org/research/mitigating-medical-misinformation-whole-society-approach-countering-spam-scams-and-hoaxes.

Kramer, Mark. 2020. "Lessons from Operation 'Denver,' the KGB's Massive AIDS Disinformation Campaign." *The MIT Press Reader.* https://thereader.mitpress.mit.edu/operation-denver-kgb-aids-disinformation-campaign/.

Rosen, Guy. 2021. "Moving Past the Finger Pointing." Facebook. https://about.fb.com/news/2021/07/support-for-covid-19-vaccines-is-high-on-facebook-and-growing/.

United Nations Children's Fund (UNICEF). 2020. *Vaccine Misinformation Management Field Guide.* https://vaccinemisinformation.guide/.

World Health Organization (WHO). n.d. "Infodemic." Accessed July 24, 2021. https://www.who.int/health-topics/infodemic-tab=tab_1.

Q27. DO CONSPIRACY THEORIES EXIST ABOUT VACCINES?

Answer: Yes. Folklore scholars and anthropologists have found that conspiracy theories are associated with many aspects of medicine, particularly in connection with infectious diseases. Many cultures have strongly held beliefs connecting purity and health, and they think of contagion as something dangerous that originates with forces outside their community. It is common in human societies for communities to blame outsiders, or corrupt insiders, for creating and transmitting the contagion during epidemics or pandemics.

During the bubonic plague pandemic of the Middle Ages, individuals and government authorities blamed both foreign enemies and marginalized peoples within their own borders for the spread of the disease, which killed nearly one-quarter of the population of Europe in the 14th century. Jews were especially targeted by these outlandish conspiracy theories, and thousands were killed by *pogroms*—massacres deliberately organized by the surrounding towns and villages. Historians have documented 351 pogroms between 1348 and 1351, as well as the destruction of over 200 Jewish communities. Of course, the theory that the Jews, or any other group of people, deliberately caused the plague was completely false and immensely tragic.

Some of the basic human beliefs and fears that fueled conspiracy theories about infection for many centuries have now been transferred to vaccination. Some conspiracy theories claim that vaccines are a kind of weapon, manufactured either by foreign powers or by scientists employed by social or political opponents. They claim that vaccines have the power to do hidden damage to DNA or fertility, thus acting, again, in the service of an individual's or community's enemies. When asked why they can provide no evidence to support any of these claims, people influenced by conspiracy theories often reply that the evidence has been covered up or suppressed by the same forces making the allegedly harmful vaccines.

Belief in conspiracy theories was behind verbal and physical attacks in West Africa on health care workers and public health officials during the Ebola clinical trials in 2014–16. They disrupted one set of trials so much that they had to be closed down, thus delaying research and preventing the development of the vaccine. Conspiracy theories that circulated in Russia and China in 2003, claiming that the SARS vaccine could damage DNA and somehow put silicon chips in the brain, resurfaced in the United States during the H1N1 epidemic in 2009. Similar theories circulated during the COVID-19 pandemic, though social media platforms took active steps to label and remove them from posts, tweets, images, and videos.

Conspiracy theories may seem odd or even funny to people who are not influenced by them. The sad truth is that they can be dangerous, especially to people who believe in them, because they keep believers from getting vaccinated and protecting themselves against infectious disease. And if conspiracists promote vaccine hesitancy or violence against health care workers, then they are also dangerous to the health and safety of everyone.

The Facts: Rumors may not seem like a medical problem, but during outbreaks they can become a serious public health problem if they decrease trust in disease prevention and treatment. This is particularly a problem in parts of the world where health care systems are fragile and where civil war and other forms of social unrest erode community trust in government actions.

The Ebola outbreak in West Africa in 2014–16 has become a model of how to develop an effective vaccine under outbreak conditions, but it has also become a cautionary tale of the role that distrust, magnified by conspiracy theories and rumors, can have in disrupting medical care. In Sierra Leone, for example, public health officials assumed as a matter of course that patients with Ebola needed to be isolated from the rest of the community. They set up a system which, on the face, of it, looked straightforward and easy to understand. The first step relied on community surveillance: anyone who became aware of someone with Ebola symptoms was to call the national hotline. Next, an ambulance would come and pick up the patient and clean the entire house with a chlorine solution. Next, the patient would be taken to a holding care center and tested for Ebola. The test took 24 hours to come back, and during that time, the patient would have to stay at the center. If patients tested positive, they'd be kept in the Ebola treatment unit. If they tested negative, they'd be released back to the community.

What was intended as an orderly process was undermined, however, by the emergence of false conspiracy theories at various stages. These included the rumor that Ebola was not a natural disease but was instead man-made to decrease the population ahead of the next presidential election. There were also rumors that patients were being suffocated by chlorine inside of ambulances and that the blood tests were really ways of stealing blood from local villages to sell on the worldwide market. These swirling conspiracy theories made people more hesitant to use the national hotline, either for fear of what might happen to sick family and neighbors, or for fear of their neighbors' anger and possible reprisals.

In sections of Guinea, "outsiders" such as politicians, journalists, and even health care workers were accused of bringing illness and manufacturing Ebola for their own purposes. Red Cross and other international health care workers were attacked and killed. The violence disrupted public health efforts and made the already devastating Ebola outbreak worse.

These conspiracy theories were later attached to clinical trials for the new Ebola vaccines. In Ghana, the nondisclosure agreements initially signed by participants led to rumors that the vaccine trials were "secret" experiments. News media spread disinformation that the clinical trials were using Ghanaian students as "guinea pigs." Other stories claimed that the trials were a way of spreading Ebola itself in Ghana. Clinical trials in Ghana finally had to be halted, showing the power of conspiracy theories to serve as disruptive forces in public health. As one report put it, "In outbreaks, rumour is the biggest killer" (Smout, 2018).

Conspiracy theories reflect the concerns of the societies that create them. During the three coronavirus epidemics (SARS, MERS, and COVID-19) in the 21st century, rumors spread that the vaccines were designed to alter DNA and insert some kind of microchip in the brain. These theories reflect concerns about the impact of genetic engineering as well as fears about the security of all the personal data people share with computers, phones, and other devices.

James Heathers, the chief scientific officer at a company that makes wearable devices to measure physiological data, used his own experience with the COVID-19 vaccine to work out why it simply isn't possible to use the vaccination process to insert any kind of microchip. "Here's what I knew," he began. He was getting the Pfizer vaccine, which came from vials, with six doses of the vaccine per vial. He estimated that the syringes being used were 25 gauge, which meant that they were half a millimeter across, with an internal diameter—that is, the width across the space inside the needle—of a quarter of a millimeter. The needle itself appeared to be about 1.5 inches long.

There were no other points of contact with health care personnel—or with anyone else. "Free hugs were neither dispensed nor encouraged. Everyone was double-masked, so an airborne microchip (were that even possible) also seemed unlikely," wrote Heathers. That meant that the only way for any microchip to be dispensed had to be through the vial or the syringe (Heathers, 2021).

What kind of microchip could fit inside such a needle? It couldn't be one with 5G functionality—the kinds that power cell phones. The smallest 5G chips as of 2021 were the size of a penny. A penny has been measured to be 19.05 millimeters in diameter. It certainly wouldn't fit inside a syringe 0.25 millimeter wide.

Even assuming that it might be possible to create a computer chip less than a quarter of a millimeter wide, how could it possibly be delivered in workable form to the inside of the human body? If it was put on the tip of the needle, then it would block the vaccine solution when the syringe pulled it upward, out of the prepackaged vial. If it was somehow imbedded within the syringe, then it might not come out when the needle was inserted into the patient.

And if this hypothetical, tiny microchip was somehow suspended in the vaccine solution, rather than being placed on the needle, then, as Heathers worked out, there would need to be at least 26 tiny devices in order to provide the greatest likelihood that each of the six doses would carry at least one. And although Heathers does not mention it, presumably a microchip would have some weight. What would keep it from sinking to the bottom of the vial? Wouldn't it be visible, at least with a microscope? Wouldn't at least some health care professionals have noticed it, as hundreds of millions of doses were distributed worldwide?

"Past a certain point," summarized Heathers, "tiny, adorable digital devices just can't scale down to having tiny, adorable batteries that make them work." Actual real medical devices are powered by "light or ultrasound that travels through the skin and is then converted into electricity," but those require some sort of very visible battery pack near the point of insertion. Any hypothetical chip that was inserted with a vaccine injection would be well below the skin, covered by layers of fat and muscle. There simply is no way to transmit electricity that far down into the human body (Heathers, 2021).

The same problem applies to how data is supposed to be extracted from the hypothetical chip. Consumers and law enforcement officials have been legitimately concerned for some time about ways that bad actors can hijack credit card information, and there are now many ways to block remote card readers. The human body, with its external layer of skin, fat, and muscle, is a natural barrier to data transmission. Our own anatomy and physiology are our own best safeguards against a hypothetical microchip (Heathers, 2021).

As conspiracy theories feed on fear, they are hard to argue against. Fear is an emotion that is entirely natural and normal during a medical crisis. In both communities and individuals, fear feeds on uncertainties and makes it hard to rationally evaluate risks, choices, and behaviors. Experts agree that the best way to deal with conspiracy theories as a public health measure is by stopping their impact as much as possible. The most effective way to do this is to implement effective social listening practices, making sure that health care professionals, teachers, and other community leaders have the training and tools to pay attention to the concerns of individuals and communities.

During the COVID-19 pandemic, conspiracy theories became another strategy for unscrupulous social media influencers to generate internet traffic or advance their own policy preferences. As the theories generated fear and confusion, they also generated more clicks than accurate information about the disease and vaccines. To remove the incentive for this kind of behavior, Twitter developed a policy against "false or misleading information." Examples of violations included statements about the "pandemic or COVID-19 vaccines that invoke a deliberate conspiracy by malicious and/or powerful forces," as well as those about "vaccines and vaccination programs which suggest that COVID-19 vaccinations are part of a deliberate or intentional attempt to cause harm or control populations" (Twitter). YouTube's COVID-19 Medical Misinformation Policy lists, and specifically prohibits, a range of false statements linked to conspiracy theories, including "claims that the COVID-19 vaccines contain a microchip or tracking device" (YouTube).

FURTHER READING

Brumfiel, Geoff. 2021. "The Life Cycle of a COVID-19 Vaccine Lie." *NPR.* https://www.npr.org/sections/health-shots/2021/07/20/1016912079/the-life-cycle-of-a-covid-19-vaccine-lie.

Heathers, James. 2021. "Putting Microchips in Vaccines Is a Terrible Idea, When You Think about It." *Atlantic.* https://www.theatlantic.com/technology/archive/2021/06/microchipped-vaccines-15-minute-investigation/619081/.

Lee, Jon. 2014. *An Epidemic of Rumors. How Stories Shape Our Perceptions of Disease.* Boulder, CO: University Press of Colorado.

Lee, Jon. 2021. "The Utter Familiarity of Even the Strangest Vaccine Conspiracy Theories." *Atlantic.* https://www.theatlantic.com/ideas/archive/2021/01/familiarity-strangest-vaccine-conspiracy-theories/617572/.

Smout, Beth, Will Schultz, and Heidi Larson. 2018. *A Guidebook on Community Engagement, Communications, and Technology for Clinical Trials in Outbreak Settings.* London: EBODAC Consortium: London School of Hygiene & Tropical Medicine. https://static1.squarespace.com/static/5d4d746d648a4e0001186e38/t/5da9a8b0da5d5c5fdd6d6f30/1571399935098/EBODAC+Guidebook-2018-06-07_v04_final.pdf.

Twitter. n.d. "COVID-19 Misleading Information Policy." Accessed August 2, 2021. https://help.twitter.com/en/rules-and-policies/medical-misinformation-policy.

YouTube. n.d. "COVID-19 Medical Misinformation Policy." Accessed August 2, 2021. https://support.google.com/youtube/answer/9891785?hl=en.

Q28. DO VACCINES CAUSE AUTISM SPECTRUM DISORDER (ASD)?

Answer: No. That claim has been completely debunked. Repeated, large-scale scientific studies have shown that there is no connection between autism spectrum disorder (ASD) and vaccines. ASD shows up in equivalent numbers in groups of children who have been vaccinated and those who have not. It is much more frequent among boys than girls, even in groups where equal numbers of boys and girls have been vaccinated.

ASD is a condition that is commonly diagnosed in children between six months to two years old. It is characterized by problems with social skills and with communication and, in severe cases, with speech and learning difficulties. As autism occurs on a spectrum of severity, cases may range from mild to severe. Early treatment can help ASD patients live happier, more productive lives.

ASD is genetic in origin, and recent scientific research focuses on connections between the disease and changes in genes that affect brain development. There is no evidence whatsoever that those genetic changes are caused either by the mother's behavior, food, drink, or medications when carrying the child or by food, drink, medication, or vaccines after the child is born.

The Facts: The idea that vaccines, specifically the measles, mumps, and rubella (MMR) vaccine, can cause autism in children has been thoroughly studied and thoroughly debunked. However, it remains a cautionary tale for how medical misinformation can be twisted into disinformation and fraud.

The term "autism" was first used in 1908 as a psychiatric category, to describe a group of patients who had been diagnosed with schizophrenia but were especially self-absorbed and withdrawn. In 1943, an American psychiatrist named Leo Kanner gave what is considered to be the first modern clinical definition of autism, based on in-depth case studies of 11 children. These children did not have any other psychiatric illness, such as schizophrenia. A year later, in Germany, Hans Asperger provided case studies of boys with similar conditions; their particular form of autism would later become known as Asperger's syndrome.

More case studies followed in the 1950s and 1960s, partly fueled by changes in how children with disabilities were cared for. Prior to World War II, children who had behavioral and learning disabilities were often sent to caretaker institutions, some of which bore names like "Home for Retarded Children." After the war, many of these institutions were closed as new ideas emerged about better ways to help disabled children live more normal lives at home and at school. Unfortunately, existing social services often lagged behind at that time. As a result, parents, teachers, and social workers stepped up and became advocates for children with behavioral challenges. They argued that children with what became known as autism spectrum disorder were not "bad" or "retarded" but rather had a medical condition that could be treated, if not cured.

Like many advocacy groups of this period, including those for patients with AIDS and many forms of cancer, ASD advocates believed that doctors were often narrow-minded in addressing their concerns. They created support networks and looked for alternative treatments. They raised awareness about environmental factors, such as contaminants in air, water, and food, that could cause or aggravate the condition of children with autism. They fought back against the idea that their children's disabilities were somehow a result of bad parenting. Finally, they lobbied local and national governments for increased access to social and medical services for people with autism.

In 1991, the U.S. government listed "autism" as a category that made children eligible for special education services. That meant that public schools had to provide appropriate educational accommodations for children with ASD, just as they did for children with other special needs. It also meant that there was a much larger pool of patients with ASD to help study and understand the condition. Other countries already had provided similar access to social services for their own ASD populations. From the 1990s on, then, there was a large body of medical and behavioral data available to researchers studying the cause and treatment of ASD.

During this same period, there were new developments in the social, political, and legal climate for vaccines. In part as a response to parent advocacy groups, pharmaceutical companies found ways to combine separate vaccines into one shot, including diphtheria, tetanus, and pertussis (DTP, later replaced by DTaP) and measles, mumps, rubella (MMR). Parents typically find bringing their very young children to be vaccinated a trying experience, as babies cry during the shot itself and may be cranky or irritable for a day or two afterward. When doses are administered together, as with the DTP and MMR vaccines, it cuts down on the number of doctor visits.

Yet some parents worried that the three-in-one shots might somehow be more dangerous than the shots to protect against single diseases. Public outcry against the vaccines flared in the United States and Europe. Pharmaceutical companies faced an upswing in lawsuits by parents alleging that the DTP vaccine caused serious adverse effects. Despite lack of scientific evidence to support these claims, large settlements were awarded in some cases. These settlements fueled additional lawsuits.

Both consumers and companies lobbied federal lawmakers for relief, claiming that the current system of trying vaccine cases in civil court was not working. Pharmaceutical companies make much less money from vaccines than from other products, and the additional cost of lawsuits led some to simply stop manufacturing vaccines. That, in turn, led to shortages and higher prices for consumers—including the U.S. government, which is a major purchaser of vaccines and related products.

Families who initiated legal action also disliked the system. Outside of some high-profile lawsuits, the awards were very limited, as it was costly and time-consuming for most families to try to prove the companies had been negligent. Even if they won a settlement, it might be much less than they had hoped for, not nearly enough to compensate them for the time, money, and emotional distress of the lawsuit.

The result was the National Vaccine Compensation Injury Program (VICP), which was established by Congress in 1986 and amended in 2016. It is administered by the U.S. Department of Health and Human Services, the U.S. Court of Federal Claims, and the U.S. Department of Justice. The VICP maintains a list of vaccines and their known adverse effects, based on medical and scientific evidence. People who believe they or their children have been adversely affected by a vaccine on the list can submit a petition or have an attorney do so on their behalf. If the adverse effect can be documented, then the compensation is awarded, without any further need for legal action.

This process spares consumers having to go to court to prove their case. However, in return for comparatively quick compensation, VICP requires that all lawsuits relating to alleged vaccine injuries have to go through its process first. That is, only after filing the petition and awaiting the VICP outcome can a consumer file a civil lawsuit against the pharmaceutical companies—and then only if they reject the VICP outcome. From 1988 through 2021, approximately $4.5 billion has been awarded in compensation.

The funding for the VICP comes from a tax placed on vaccine manufacturers of 75 cents per dose of vaccine. For pharmaceutical companies, the price is well worth the result, which has been to cut down significantly on the number of civil lawsuits. The results of the VICP petitions are also considered to be "no fault," that is, they do not imply negligence on the part of the company manufacturing the vaccine. If a petition is successful, and a parent or child is awarded compensation for adverse effects from vaccination, it doesn't mean that the company manufacturing the vaccine has been found to be at fault. In other words, the VICP did not make companies more liable for additional lawsuits.

Though largely successful, the VICP did have certain vulnerabilities, particularly in its early years. The main one was that the criteria for what counted as "adverse effects" was not always based on science or medicine. As the original purpose of the program was to cut down on lawsuits, some adverse effects were compensated, not because they had been scientifically proven but rather because they had appeared in many lawsuits. For example, petitions for adverse effects from the DTP vaccine were much more likely to be compensated in the first few years of the VICP than they would be today because of the publicity that surrounded so many of the early lawsuits. The lawmakers who created the program believed this would allow petitioners, some of whom had already spent years in court, to be compensated "quickly, easily, and with certainty and generosity" (Hamblin, 2019).

One unintended consequence was to create the impression that consumer-based complaints against pharmaceutical companies were an acceptable way to document adverse effects. Another was to suggest that any researcher who could find a smoking gun that proved that vaccines caused adverse effects could end up rich and famous.

In the early 1990s, the rumors about DTP had largely died down, but similar concerns had begun to spread about MMR. In particular, rumors began circulating in Great Britain among parents of children with ASD that the MMR vaccine might be responsible. Several families contacted a lawyer, Richard Barr, who had been involved in high-profile lawsuits against pharmaceutical companies. He, in turn, contacted the Legal Services Commission, a government program that provides legal aid, to obtain funds for research. The law firm received an amount equivalent to $30 million—$20 million to pay for legal fees and $10 million to doctors and scientists. There was a clear assumption that the money would be spent on research that supported the lawsuit, rather than any that undermined it.

The most notorious of the scientists employed by Barr's lawsuit was Andrew Wakefield., who received more than $800,000 to carry out research in support of Barr's claim. Wakefield's 1998 article, "Heal-lymphoid-nodular Hyperplasia, Non-Specific Colitis, and Pervasive Developmental Disorder in Children," claimed to show a direct, causal link between the MMR vaccine and autism.

In reality, however, Wakefield engaged in a classic example of scientific fraud. There were only 12 children in the study, and they were chosen because their symptoms best fit the hypothesis Wakefield wanted to prove. Several of the families were parties in Barr's lawsuit—something that should have disqualified them for taking part in any impartial scientific study. The actual data provided in the article was false as well. In fact, the data was literally made up to "prove" the connection between MMR and ASD. At no point did Wakefield reveal the sources of his funding or reveal obvious conflicts of interest. He also did not wait for scientific replication of his initial "findings," which were published in the prestigious journal the *Lancet*. Instead, he announced them at a press conference, to instant public acclaim.

Wakefield's frauds were later exposed, however, and he had his medical license revoked in Great Britain. Many of his associates were also shown to have accepted large sums from the Legal Services Commission grant and to have used the money to carry out research that was later discredited. The *Lancet* was criticized by other medical and scientific journals for not subjecting the Wakefield article to thorough peer review, which would have revealed the shoddy research. The press was criticized as well for having accepted Wakefield's announcement without doing any fact-checking.

Over the next 10 years, study after scientific study worldwide showed not only the failures of Wakefield's own research but also the complete lack of evidence to connect MMR and ASD. The same results came back from the legal system when the VICP took up the case. Over 5,300 petitions alleging a connection between MMR and autism had been filed by 2002. The VICP agreed to consider them under the Omnibus Autism Proceeding, in which the six strongest cases, with the most evidence, were presented before judges appointed by the Court of Federal Claims. In 2009 they handed down their decision: there was no causal connection between the MMR vaccine and ASD. Since that time, the VICP has routinely denied petitions for compensation that claim the connection exists.

Reputable ASD advocacy groups today all recommend standard immunizations for children. Children and adults with ASD have the opportunity to be as physically healthy as other individuals, and they have the right to the same protection against vaccine-preventable diseases.

FURTHER READING

Hamblin, James. 2019. "Why the Government Pays Billions to People Who Claim Injury by Vaccines." *Atlantic*. https://www.theatlantic.com /health/archive/2019/05/vaccine-safety-program/589354/.

Health Resources and Services Administration. n.d. "National Vaccine Injury Compensation Program." Accessed August 4, 2021. https://www .hrsa.gov/vaccine-compensation/index.html.

"History of Anti-vaccination Movements." n.d. *History of Vaccines*. Accessed August 4, 2021. https://ftp.historyofvaccines.org/multilanguage/content /articles/history-anti-vaccination-movements.

Hviid, Anders, Jorgen Hansen, Morten Frisch, and Mads Melbye. 2019. "Measles, Mumps, Rubella Vaccination and Autism." *Annals of Internal Medicine* 170 (8). https://www.acpjournals.org/doi/10.7326/m18-2101.

Offit, Paul. 2008. *Autism's False Prophets. Bad Science, Risky Medicine, and the Search for a Cure.* New York: Columbia University Press.

Q29. CAN VACCINATION BE MADE COMPULSORY?

Answer: That depends. Many countries have legal mechanisms that would allow governments to make vaccinations compulsory. However, there would be huge practical barriers to passing laws that would require everyone to be vaccinated. Most governments that tried to force vaccination on every single person would face legal and political challenges. Enforcement of a vaccination mandate could be as difficult as enforcing the laws that require everyone to wear seatbelts.

In the 21st century, the right of a person to control his/her/their own health and body is considered a fundamental human right by the United Nations. Though formulated originally to protect people against bodily harm—such as rape and torture—that right is also understood as including the right to refuse health care. During the COVID-19 pandemic, even countries willing to use government power to impose strict lockdowns and other quarantine measure did not impose national vaccine mandates on every single person in the country.

Many institutions and employers do have the legal authority to make vaccinations compulsory as a condition of a person's continued affiliation or employment. Moreover, national, regional, and local governments can create regulations that encourage compliance. For example, public and private schools and universities have a long history of requiring students, faculty, and staff to be vaccinated as a public health measure. This is because children and young adults are especially vulnerable to vaccine-preventable diseases, and clusters of unvaccinated children can lead to outbreaks in both schools and wider communities. Health care facilities also have long histories of requiring certain vaccines in order to protect patients and staff alike.

Businesses can also require proof of vaccination, in the same way they can set dress codes and decide "No shirt, no shoes, no service." Once COVID-19 vaccines were widely available, many restaurants, theaters, concert halls, and other public entertainment venues required employees and patrons to be vaccinated. Entry signs with "No shot, no shoes, no service" and similar messages became common in many locations.

In their capacity as employers, national, regional, and local governments can require their own employees to be vaccinated. They can also pass and enforce public health ordinances to require public venues to check for proof of vaccination before admitting customers. France, Italy, and Israel all enacted regulations to require COVID-19 vaccination for virtually all public venues. In the United States, the federal government and some states, such as New York, passed similar legislation.

These regulations have been criticized by some unvaccinated people, who viewed them as discriminatory. However, lawsuits that challenged vaccination requirements came up against the legal reality that employers have wide authority for regulating their own employees. In most places, the same authority that allows them to require background checks, enforce dress codes, and monitor email also gives them the authority to require proof of vaccination.

Employers or institutions that require vaccination do not violate the legal or human rights of their staff, customers, clients, or students, because people have a free choice as to whether they wish to take a particular job, visit a particular gym, or attend a particular school. If they do not want to be vaccinated, they can choose to go elsewhere.

In the United States, employers or institutions that require vaccination are, in turn, required to allow exemptions for employees with disabilities or those who have religious objections. Employees who are exempted from the vaccination requirement may be required to undergo ongoing testing and to observe social distancing measures.

The Facts: For most of their history, compulsory vaccines have been controversial. However, national, state, regional, and local jurisdictions, whatever their political divisions in other areas, have tended to support them, because the public health and economic consequences of allowing infectious diseases to spread is so dangerous.

Within the United States, laws and regulations that make up public health policy are divided among federal, state, and local governments. Though the federal government can do a great deal to develop and distribute vaccines, it has limited power to compel people to take them. It can require vaccines for its own employees, at home and abroad, and it can also regulate vaccine requirements that affect interstate commerce and travel across national borders. But it has no political or legal authority to compel individuals to get vaccinated, or to require private businesses to make vaccination compulsory for employees or customers. This is in contrast to other countries, such as France, Italy, and Israel, where national governments do have the political and legal power to require vaccination for schools, businesses, and recreational facilities.

Federal laws can have an impact in other, less direct ways. Federal law determines what kinds of categories can be used by the U.S. Equal Employment Opportunity Commission (EEOC) in lawsuits involving alleged job discrimination. The EEOC "is responsible for enforcing federal laws that make it illegal to discriminate against a job applicant or an employee because of the person's race, color, religion, sex (including pregnancy, transgender status, and sexual orientation), national origin, age (40 or older), disability or genetic information." These laws apply to workplaces with more than 15 employees and are incorporated into union agreements as well (EEOC, 2021). They are important for the legal standing of vaccine mandates because "vaccination status"—that is, whether or not a person has been vaccinated—has never been a category enforceable by the EEOC. What that means is that private businesses can require vaccines for all employees without being investigated, fined, or sued in federal court for discriminatory hiring practices.

Individual states do have the power to require individuals to be vaccinated. The legal case that set the precedent for this was *Jacobson v. the State of Massachusetts*, from 1905. At that time, Massachusetts was one of only 11 states that had laws in place allowing local public health authorities to require smallpox vaccination for adults 21 and older, if they felt it was necessary for the health and safety of the community. Those who refused were subject to a $5 fine.

Henning Jacobson, a pastor in Cambridge, Massachusetts, in the early 1900s, felt he and his family had a hereditary condition that made smallpox vaccination dangerous for them. He refused to be vaccinated or pay the fine. Jacobson argued that "his liberty is invaded when the state subjects him to fine or imprisonment for neglecting or refusing to submit to vaccination" and "that a compulsory vaccination law is unreasonable, arbitrary, and oppressive, and, therefore, hostile to the inherent right of every freeman to care for his own body and health" (Beck, 2021).

The Massachusetts Supreme Court disagreed, arguing that Jacobson's case was already covered under the existing statute: "If a person should deem it important that vaccination should not be performed in his case, and the authorities should think otherwise, it is not in their power to vaccinate him by force, and the worst that could happen to him under the statute would be the payment of $5" (Mariner, 2005).

Jacobson appealed his case to the Supreme Court, which ruled against him, 7-2, and provided the precedents for current decisions on vaccine mandates at the state and local level. The Supreme Court decision in

Jacobson v. the State of Massachusetts stated clearly that a compulsory vaccination law is not "unreasonable, arbitrary, and oppressive." Instead, it may become a necessary part of a state government's responsibility for preserving the health and safety of its citizens. According to the decision, "[T]he liberty secured by the Constitution of the United States to every person within its jurisdiction does not import an absolute right in each person to be, at all times and in all circumstances, wholly freed from restraint. There are manifold restraints to which every person is necessarily subject for the common good. On any other basis organized society could not exist with safety to its members. Society based on the rule that each one is a law unto himself would soon be confronted with disorder and anarchy."

In particular, legal arguments that "attach little or no value to vaccination as a means of preventing" disease, or that claim "that vaccination causes other diseases," were not valid in court. Courts had to be based on the best scientific information available, and "the common belief . . . is that [vaccination] has a decided tendency to prevent the spread" of smallpox "and to render it less dangerous to those who contract it. While not accepted by all, it is accepted by the mass of the people, as well as by most members of the medical profession. It has been general . . . in most civilized nations for generations. It is generally accepted in theory, and generally applied in practice, both by the voluntary action of the people, and in obedience to the command of law." The Supreme Court therefore concluded "We are not prepared to hold that a minority, residing or remaining in any [place] where [an epidemic disease] is prevalent, and enjoying the general protection afforded by an organized local government, may thus defy the will of its constituted authorities" (Beck, 2021).

While *Jacobson v. the State of Massachusetts* established the legal precedent for state and local governments to enact legislation requiring vaccination, it also established the key exemption. The Supreme Court decision concluded, "We are not inclined to hold that the statute establishes the absolute rule that an adult must be vaccinated if it be apparent or can be shown with reasonable certainty that he is not at the time a fit subject of vaccination or that vaccination, by reason of his then condition, would seriously impair his health or probably cause his death" (Mosvick, 2021). This aspect of the case has been incorporated into modern medical and religious exemptions found in most vaccine requirements.

The power of public schools and universities to require vaccination has also been tested in court. In 2021, eight students brought a lawsuit against Indiana University's requirement that, starting in fall 2021, all students must be vaccinated against COVID-19 unless they are exempt for medical or religious reasons. While waiting for that suit to go to trial, they filed a motion in federal court asking for a preliminary injunction to override the requirement. The judges ruled against the injunction, citing *Jacobson v. the State of Massachusetts* as the applicable law, which allowed compulsory vaccination. They pointed out that students who did not wish to be vaccinated could study at other universities, and that there was no constitutional right to study at any particular university. "Each university," the judges noted, "may decide to do what is necessary to keep students safe in a congregate setting. Health exams and vaccinations against other diseases (measles, mumps, rubella, diphtheria, pertussis, tetanus, varicella, meningitis, influenza, and more) are common requirements of higher education. Vaccination protects not only the vaccinated person, but also those who come into contact with them, and at a university close contact is inevitable" (*Klassen v. Trustees of Indiana University*, 2021).

Private employers can also require vaccination. In fact, they may be required to, if not doing so would put their employees or customers at risk. According to the federal Occupational Safety and Health Act (OSHA), employers have to provide an environment free from known health and safety hazards, including the likelihood of catching vaccine-preventable diseases. Under this provision, if infectious disease would pose a serious health hazard, employers can require vaccination. During the COVID-19 pandemic, for example, many cruise lines required everyone onboard their ships, including crew members and passengers, to have received COVID-19 vaccines. This followed the devastating outbreaks early in the pandemic on more than 40 cruise ships, resulting in thousands of cases and hundreds of deaths.

FURTHER READING

Beck, James M. 2021. "Survival of the Vaxxest." 2021. *Drug and Device Law.* https://www.druganddevicelawblog.com/2021/08/survival-of-the-vaxxest .html.

Cohen, Roger. 2021. "Persuasion vs. Coercion: Vaccine Debate in Europe Heats Up." *New York Times.* https://www.nytimes.com/2021/07/23/world /europe/france-covid-vaccine-coercion.html.

Klaassen v. Trustees of Indiana University, 7th U.S. Circuit Court of Appeals, No. 21-2326. https://media.ca7.uscourts.gov/cgi-bin/rssExec.pl?Submit= Display&Path=Y2021/D08-02/C:21-2326:J:Easterbrook:aut:T:op:N:274175 3:S:0.

Kostov, Nick, and Eric Sylvers. 2021. "France, Italy Require Proof of Covid-19 Status for Restaurants, Bars." *Wall Street Journal.* https://www.wsj .com/articles/france-italy-require-health-pass-restaurants-bars -11628587800.

Lomas, Natasha. 2021. "EU's COVID-19 'Digital Pass' Gateway System Goes Live." *TechCrunch*. https://techcrunch.com/2021/06/01/eus-covid -19-digital-pass-gateway-system-goes-live/.

Mariner, Wendy, George Annas, and Leonard Glanz. 2005. "*Jacobson v. Massachusetts*: It's Not Your Great-Great-Grandfather's Public Health Law." *American Journal of Public Health* 95 (4): 581–90. https://ajph .aphapublications.org/doi/10.2105/AJPH.2004.055160.

Mosvick, Nicholas. 2021. "On This Day, the Supreme Court Rules on Vaccines and Public Health." *Constitution Daily, National Constitution Center.* https://constitutioncenter.org/blog/on-this-day-the-supreme-court-rules -on-vaccines-and-public-health.

United States Equal Employment Opportunity Commission (EEOC). n.d. "Overview." Accessed August 11, 2021. https://www.eeoc.gov/overview.

Q30. CAN TEENAGERS GET VACCINATED WITHOUT PARENTAL CONSENT?

Answer: That depends. Throughout the world, people aged 18 and above are considered to be legally adults. That means that they can choose to be vaccinated, even if their parents don't approve.

For people under 18, though, both law and practice vary from country to country, and often from region to region. In France, the age of consent is 18 and above. In Canada and the United Kingdom, the age of consent for vaccinations is 16 and above in many districts, with some allowing younger teens to self-consent. Within the United States, the youngest age of vaccination consent is 10 and up, in Philadelphia, and 11 and up, in the District of Columbia. In Alabama, the age of consent is 14 and up; in Oregon, 15 and up; and in South Carolina, 16 and up. Five states follow what is called the "mature minor doctrine," which allows minors to make their own health care decisions as long as their health care provider believes they are capable of making an informed decision. These states are North Carolina, Tennessee, Arkansas, Washington, and Idaho.

Before giving any vaccine to minors, whether or not their parents are present, health care providers must be sure that they are capable of informed consent. Scientists who study brain development have found that from the age of 14 or so forward, teen decision-making tracks that of adults when it comes to medical matters. That is, teens from the age of about 14 are fully capable of understanding the benefits and potential risks of vaccines and can make decisions about what is best for them.

In Canada, the nation's Supreme Court has ruled that teenagers who are "mature minors" should have the same control over their own bodies, with the same right to accept or decline health care, as those who are legally adults. The United States, with its patchwork of jurisdictions, does not have a single policy that applies everywhere.

The Facts: Health care providers involved with adolescent patients often run into questions about whether teens, or their parents, should make important health care questions. This is especially the case when teens may have questions about sensitive subjects such as sex, sexually transmitted diseases, or pregnancy, but don't want their parents to know. Usually, health care providers want to treat teens as decision makers and respect their privacy and autonomy, but local laws may require them to give priority to the parents' views and require their consent.

Debates about whether teens should be able to get vaccinated without parental approval have intensified in the 21st century because new vaccines were developed that are best given during adolescence. These included vaccines for meningitis and human papillomavirus (HPV). All health care providers agreed that infants and young children could not make their own decisions about vaccination. However, many who worked with adolescents felt that they were just as capable of making informed decisions as their parents. Many argued that adolescents should be encouraged to educate themselves, so they can make their own decisions and become their own best health care advocates.

These issues received a boost of publicity in 2017 when high school senior Ethan Lindenberger turned to social media to ask an unusual question: where could he go to get ordinary childhood vaccines like measles, mumps, and polio? His mother was extremely fearful about vaccines, with the result that neither he nor his younger brothers and sisters had ever been vaccinated. His public school had state-mandated vaccine requirements. However, as he later explained, "In school, I was pulled out of class every year and told that if I did not receive my shots, I wouldn't be able to attend my high school. But, every year, I was opted out of these immunizations," as his state allowed parents to claim medical and religious exemptions from the vaccine requirements. "Because of current legislation," Lindenberger said, "I was allowed to attend a public high school despite placing my classmates in danger of contracting multiple preventable diseases" (Lindenberger, 2019). And not only his classmates: Ethan recognized that he could be putting his own family in danger as well.

The reaction, both positive and negative, to his posts led Lindenberger to become a vaccination advocate, for his own sake and for teens like him who disagreed with their parents' anti-vaccination views. His story was picked up by national and international media. He received numerous invitations to speak, including noteworthy appearances at the United Nations and before the United States Senate Committee on Health, Education, Welfare, and Pensions.

In his testimony to the Senate, Lindenberger began by sharing some of his family background. "I grew up understanding that my mother believed vaccines are dangerous," he said, "as she would speak openly about her views both online and in person. These beliefs were met with strong criticism, and over the course of my life seeds of doubt were planted and questions arose because of the backlash my mother received when sharing her views on vaccines" (Lindenberger, 2019).

At first, Lindenberger had only minor concerns, but as he entered high school, he began to look at his mother's views with a more critical eye. He explained that he "ran a debate club and learned about the importance of finding credible information both through my own pursuits in leading this club and through the fantastic teachers at Norwalk." Among the lessons he learned was that "to find credible research and information is fundamental to finding truth in a world of misleading facts and false views." Through leading his debate club, he "saw there are almost universally two or more sides to every discussion. To every claim there is a counterclaim, and to every statement there was always a rebuttal" (Lindenberger, 2019).

Yet when it came to vaccines, that claim and counterclaim didn't work. Lindenberger carried out his own careful research, using the Centers for Disease Control and Prevention (CDC) and World Health Organization (WHO) websites and resources. He found that "scientific studies and evidence that analyze the benefits and risk of vaccinations" were completely convincing. "In its essence, there is no debate. Vaccinations are proven to be a medical miracle, stopping the spread of numerous diseases and therefore saving countless lives" (Lindenberger, 2019).

At that point, Lindenberger decided to catch up on all the childhood vaccines that he had missed. As he was under 18, he began by discussing his views with his mother. As he later told the congressional committee, he found the experience very frustrating. As an example, "at one point in our discussion she claimed a link existed between vaccines and autism. In response, I presented evidence from the CDC which claimed directly in large bold letters, 'There is no link between vaccines and autism.' Within the same article from the CDC on their official website, extensive evidence and studies from the institute of medicine (IOM) were cited. Most would assume when confronted with such strong proof, there would be serious consideration that your views are incorrect. This was not the case for my mother, as her only response was, 'that's what they want you to think.'" As he noted, "And this response is representative of the entire discussion around vaccines, where one side is based in scientific evidence and truth while the other is based in skepticism and falsities" (Lindenberger, 2019).

Initially, Lindenberger was angry at his mother for preventing him from being vaccinated. His first posts, which he later regretted, described her views as "kind of stupid." But he later apologized for that, trying to separate out the misinformation—which he continued to think was stupid—from the person delivering it. As he emphasized to the congressional committee, "anti-vaccine parents and individuals are in no way evil." What was evil, in Lindenberger's view, was "anti-vaccine leaders and proponents of misinformation," especially those online, "which knowingly lie to the American people." While trying to keep a "tone of respectful disagreement" in his conversations with his mother, Lindenberger was very critical of the people she listened to. "Using the love, affection, and care of a parent for their children to push an agenda and create false distress is shameful. The sources which spread misinformation should be the primary concern of the American people," as well as the congressional committee to which he was speaking. He hoped his testimony, social media platforms, and Congress would work to shut down all those sources of misinformation. Using "a parent's love as a tool," he said, "these lies cause people to distrust in vaccination, furthering the impact of a preventable disease outbreak and even contributing to the cause of diseases spreading" (Lindenberger, 2019).

During the COVID-19 pandemic, many teens found that their own experiences mirrored Lindenberger's. The Pfizer vaccine received Emergency Use Authorization for adolescents 12 years and up on May 20, 2021, and many teens looked forward to the freedom it would bring. But teens whose parents did not approve could not get the vaccine unless they lived in one of the few jurisdictions that allowed them to self-consent.

Teens whose parents wouldn't allow them to get the shot found themselves excluded from social gatherings. "Five of my friends are throwing a party and they invited me," said one 15-year-old, "but then they said, 'Are you vaccinated?'" she said. "So I can't go. That hurts." Her friends posted their vaccination status on social media, "and now when I see them, they ask me things like, 'Where have you been? Are you traveling a lot? Are you sure you don't have Covid?' It sucks that I can't get the shot," she said (Hoffman, 2021).

To provide information for teens who wanted the COVID-19 vaccine, but whose parents did not approve, high school senior Kelly Danielpour founded VaxTeen.org, a website that provides authoritative information about vaccination. It has a teen-friendly user interface and provides links to vaccine consent laws, by state. It also provides links to guides for CDC-recommended vaccines. VaxTeen's mission is to reverse "the decline in vaccinations by encouraging teens and young adults to take responsibility for their own health." The website was designed to communicate "directly with teenagers and young adults to counter this dangerous tide of misinformation, encouraging those who are unvaccinated to catch up on vaccines as soon as they can by helping them find out what immunizations they need and how they can get them" (VaxTeen, 2021).

Public health experts recommend that even with so many opportunities for disagreement, children and parents should try to keep channels of communication open. VeryWell Health developed an interactive Conversation Coach to help people have more productive conversations with vaccine skeptics. It allows users to choose among several options for their part in the conversation, and it explains why certain responses are better than others. The best ones are those that are least confrontational and provide more opportunities to debunk false or misleading information (Spiegel, 2021).

Whatever the law, teens who live at home with their parents may have a hard time going against their parents' wishes when it comes to vaccination. Websites such as VaxTeen (https://www.vaxteen.org/how-to-talk-to-your-parents) provide helpful suggestions on how teens can talk to parents about getting vaccines against COVID-19 or other vaccine-preventable diseases. Nemours Children's Hospital has useful information on how older teens can take charge of their own medical care (https://kidshealth.org/en/teens/medical-care.html-cathealth-basics).

FURTHER READING

Downshen, Stephen. 2018. "Taking Charge of Your Medical Care." *TeensHealth from Nemours*. https://kidshealth.org/en/teens/medical-care.html-cathealth-basics.

Hoffman, Jan. 2021. "As Parents Forbid Covid Shots, Defiant Teenagers Seek Ways to Get Them." *New York Times*. https://www.nytimes.com/2021/06/26/health/covid-vaccine-teens-consent.html.

Lindenberger, Ethan. 2019. United States Senate. Committee on Health, Education, Welfare, and Pensions. "Vaccines Save Lives: What Is Driving Preventable Disease Outbreaks?" https://www.help.senate.gov/hearings/vaccines-save-lives-what-is-driving-preventable-disease-outbreaks.

Morgan, Larissa, Jason Schwartz, Dominic Sisti. 2021. "COVID-19 Vaccination of Minors without Parental Consent. Respecting Emerging

Autonomy and Advancing Public Health." *Journal of the American Medical Association Pediatrics.* https://jamanetwork.com/journals/jamapediatrics/fullarticle/2782024.

Singer, Natalie, Jennifer Kates, Jennifer Tolbert. 2021. "COVID-19 Vaccination and Parental Consent." *Kaiser Family Foundation (KFF).* https://www.kff.org/policy-watch/covid-19-vaccination-and-parental-consent/.

Spiegel, Brett. 2021. "How to Talk to a Vaccine Skeptic." *VeryWell Health.* https://www.verywellhealth.com/how-to-talk-to-a-vaccine-skeptic-4590366.

VaxTeen. n.d. "Young People Taking Responsibility for Their Own Health to Put an End to Preventable Diseases." Accessed August 22, 2021. https://www.vaxteen.org/.

Q31. CAN VACCINATION BE REQUIRED IN HEALTH CARE SETTINGS?

Answer: That depends. In the United States, health care organizations such as hospitals and clinics can require vaccinations for their employees, though some allow exemptions for medical, religious, and philosophical reasons. During the COVID-19 pandemic, many health care facilities required all employees to be vaccinated. Although employee advocates sued, the courts upheld the rights of the employees to require vaccination in order to protect the health of patients and other employees.

For patients, the rules are more complicated. Health care providers that receive federal or state funding generally cannot refuse any patient, including those who are not vaccinated. The only exceptions might be for patients who might put themselves, or others, in immediate danger if they were not vaccinated. For example, a patient who might be at risk for Ebola and who refused the Ebola vaccine could legitimately be refused entry to any health care facility. However, in most cases, the risk of vaccine-preventable disease is not that high. So a patient who needed an appendectomy, for example, but who had not received childhood vaccinations or a flu shot could not be refused admission to a hospital for that reason.

Private medical practices can legally refuse to treat patients who have not been vaccinated, though ethical questions may remain. This has primarily been an issue for pediatric practices. Pediatricians routinely administer childhood vaccines, and most parents follow their judgment in vaccination as in other aspects of their children's health care. However, pediatricians have seen an increase in the number of vaccine-hesitant parents. Around 87 percent of pediatricians say that they have had conversations with parents in their practice who are vaccine-hesitant or who refuse vaccination for their children.

This situation is challenging for pediatricians, as unvaccinated children are vulnerable to outbreaks of vaccine-preventable diseases. A number of vaccines require more than one shot to be fully effective, and until children have received the all the shots, they are not completely protected. They may still contract the disease if they come into contact with an unvaccinated child who carries it. Pediatricians want to be sure that their office does not become the point of contact for an outbreak.

During measles outbreaks in the United States and Canada, for example, epidemiologists found that the disease spread first to unvaccinated children who brought it back from travels overseas. From them, measles spread to communities with a reservoir of unvaccinated children. From those children, the disease spread to very young children who had only received the first shot, as the second is usually given between the ages of four and six. It also passed to children and adults who were *immunocompromised*; that is, people with immune systems that are not as effective in forming antibodies to repel infectious diseases.

Due to concerns over these and other outbreaks, surveys have found that around 40 percent of pediatricians have considered dismissing families from their practices who will not agree to be vaccinated. This is a very difficult decision for pediatricians, who specifically chose to work with children in order to help protect and treat them. Many are concerned that if they refuse to accept into their practice children whose parents won't vaccinate them, those children will be doubly put at risk. And yet, as the number of cases of measles and other vaccine-preventable diseases has risen alarmingly, some pediatricians have come to believe that their primary responsibility is to protect the other children who receive care in their practice.

The Facts: Health care facilities have had mandatory vaccination requirements for many years. The most common requirement is for tetanus vaccines, which are generally required even for volunteers. Full-time staff are often required to have influenza vaccines as well as the standard vaccines recommended for early childhood and adolescence. Studies have shown that health care facilities that require influenza vaccines have fewer outbreaks and overall better health care records than those that do not.

The reasoning behind the vaccine requirements is simple: the vaccines protect both patients and the rest of the staff. Under the federal Occupational Health and Safety Act (OSHA) as well as many state and local laws, employers have an obligation to provide a workplace that is free from known occupational hazards. If the workplace is a children's hospital, for example, it is an occupational hazard that patients may come in with vaccine-preventable diseases. If it is a respiratory unit in an urban or rural hospital or a nursing facility for older patients, then it is an occupational hazard that patients may be admitted with influenza. It is therefore reasonable for those employers to require vaccination because it protects both the patients the facility is designed to serve and the people who work there.

OSHA is not the only applicable law, however. Health care facilities also have to pay attention to the Equal Employment Opportunity Commission (EEOC), which has identified two types of exemptions to mandatory vaccination requirements. The first is for employees with certain disabilities that make it dangerous for them to receive the vaccine. This could be for a condition that has left them immunocompromised or for an allergy to some product used in the vaccine in question. The EEOC also recommends that pregnant women be exempt from vaccine requirements. The second exemption is for employees who have religious beliefs that prevent them from being vaccinated. In past lawsuits, courts have interpreted "religious beliefs" broadly. For example, in one case an employee who was vegan was exempted from having to take a vaccine made using chicken eggs.

During the COVID-19 pandemic, the legal status of mandatory vaccine requirements in health care settings came up early in the vaccine rollout. In March 2021, two months after the COVID-19 vaccines were available for health care workers, Houston Methodist Hospital in Houston, Texas, required all 26,000 employees either to get the COVID-19 vaccine, request an exemption or deferral, or have their employment terminated.

The policy was first announced on March 31, with all managers required to get at least the first shot of the available vaccines by April 15. There was high compliance with this policy, and 99 percent of managers met the deadline. The next step was for the rest of the employees to comply with the policy by June 7. At that time, Houston Methodist reported almost 100 percent compliance. A spokesman for the hospital said, "Our employees and physicians made their decisions for our patients, who are always at the center of everything we do" (Kaplan, 2021).

However, 178 of the Houston Methodist health care system's 26,000 employees refused to comply with the policy; they were placed on suspension, and those that continued to refuse vaccination were terminated. Among the terminated employees were 112 individuals who filed a lawsuit to block the injections as well as the terminations. The plaintiffs argued that the hospital acted unlawfully in forcing their employees to either be vaccinated or be fired. The hospital, in turn, moved that the lawsuit be dismissed.

The judge agreed with the hospital and dismissed the lawsuit. According to the decision, the plaintiffs spent the bulk of the complaint arguing "that the currently available COVID-19 vaccines are experimental and dangerous." However, the judge stated, "This claim is false, and it is also irrelevant." The plaintiffs argued that if they were to be fired for refusing the vaccine, they would be wrongfully terminated. But Texas law is very specific: the only basis for a wrongful termination lawsuit is if the employer asks the employee to carry out an illegal act that carries legal penalties. However, "Receiving a COVID-19 vaccination is not an illegal act, and it carries no criminal penalties."

The hospital was, in fact, following all appropriate legal and policy guidance. Vaccine mandates were clearly consistent with federal and state legal precedent. The EEOC had issued guidance that COVID-19 vaccine mandates should be allowed, as long as reasonable accommodation was made for employees with medical or religious exemptions. The plaintiffs, unlike the rest of the employees, were "refusing to accept inoculation that, in the hospital's judgment, will make it safer for their workers and the patients in Methodist's care."

To the argument made by the claimants that they were being coerced into getting the COVID-19 vaccine for fear of being fired, the judge responded, "This is not coercion. Methodist is trying to do their business of saving lives without giving them the COVID-19 virus. It is a choice made to keep staff, patients, and their families safer." Employers have every legal right to establish conditions of employment for their employees and to dismiss those employees who do not fulfill those conditions. The plaintiffs were free "to accept or refuse a COVID-19 vaccine." However, if they refuse, they "will simply need to work somewhere else. If a worker refuses an assignment, changed office, earlier start time, or other directive, he may be properly fired. Every employment includes limits on the worker's behavior in exchange for his remuneration. That is all part of the bargain" (U.S. District Court, 2021).

Once full FDA approval was granted for the COVID-19 vaccines, many health care facilities made it mandatory for all employees. But others did not, often because they already faced shortages of nursing and other skilled health care staff. Even without vaccine requirements, health care facilities were not unsafe. They retained the procedures they put into effect in the early months of the pandemic.

Although the legal system allows employers to require employees to be vaccinated, there is no provision anywhere that requires patients to be vaccinated when they visit a doctor. For most health care settings, the question doesn't arise. Any patients, suffering from any illness, can expect to go to see a doctor or visit a clinic or an emergency room and be treated regardless of vaccine status.

One area where that may not be true is in the offices of pediatricians in private practice. As the number of vaccine-refusing parents increased, so has the number of pediatricians who believe that it might be the right decision to ask them to leave their practice. They note that the parents' decision not to vaccinate their own child puts other children in the practice at risk. They further note that many of the reasons given for vaccine refusal are not based on sound science. Finally, some pediatricians assert that if the pediatrician and the parents disagree so much on the value of vaccination, then they are unlikely to see eye to eye on other health care decisions made by the parents for their children.

For many years, the American Academy of Pediatrics (AAP) advised against dismissing parents, arguing that it was better to retain them in the practice and attempt to convince them of the value of vaccination. However, surveys of pediatricians showed that if parents continued to refuse to accept vaccines, physicians could do little to change their minds. In fact, in some cases, the suggestion that the parents leave the practice turned out to be the key that convinced them that their children should be vaccinated.

The AAP revised the guidelines in 2016 in response to surveys from the group's membership. The new guidelines stated that in some cases, and as a last resort, physicians may make the ethical decision to dismiss those who consistently refuse vaccines from their practice. "The decision to dismiss a family who continues to refuse immunization is not one that should be made lightly," the guidelines state, "nor should it be made without considering and respecting the reasons for the parents' point of view. Nevertheless, the individual pediatrician may consider dismissal of families who refuse vaccination as an acceptable option. In all practice settings, consistency, transparency, and openness regarding the practice's policy on vaccines is important" (Edwards, 2016).

FURTHER READING

Block, Stan. 2015. "The Pediatrician's Dilemma: Refusing the Refusers of Infant Vaccines." *Journal of Law, Medicine & Ethics* 43 (3): 648–53. https://www.cambridge.org/core/journals/journal-of-law-medicine-and-ethics/article/abs/pediatricians-dilemma-refusing-the-refusers-of-infant-vaccines/50D4F7B518D54ED76CDE6D05BF5A275A.

Edwards, Kathryn, and Jesse M. Hackell. 2016. "Countering Vaccine Hesitancy. The Committee on Infectious Diseases, the Committee on Practice and

Ambulatory Medicine." *Pediatrics* 138(3): e20162146. https://pediatrics
.aappublications.org/content/138/3/e20162146.

Field, Robert. 2009. "Mandatory Vaccination of Health Care Workers:
Whose Rights Should Come First?" *P & T: A peer-reviewed journal for
formulary management* 34 (1): 615–18. https://www.ncbi.nlm.nih.gov
/pmc/articles/PMC2810172/.

Hough-Telford, Catherine, David Kimberlin, Inmaculada Aban, William
Hitchcock, Jon Almquist, Richard Kratz, and Karen O'Connor. 2016.
"Vaccine Delays, Refusals, and Patient Dismissals: A Survey of Pediatricians." *Pediatrics* 138 (3) (2016): e20162127. https://pediatrics.aappublica
tions.org/content/138/3/e20162127.

Kaplan, Sheila. 2021. "A Judge Dismisses Houston Hospital Workers' Lawsuit about Vaccine Mandates." *New York Times.* https://www.nytimes
.com/2021/06/13/health/houston-hospital-vaccine-mandate-lawsuit
.html.

United States District Court Southern District of Texas. 2021. "21-1774—
Bridges, et al. v. Houston Methodist Hospital et al." Government.
Administrative Office of the United States Courts, June 11, 2021. https://
docs.justia.com/cases/federal/district-courts/texas/txsdce/4:202
1cv01774/1830373/18.

Q32. CAN CONSUMERS BRING LEGAL ACTION AGAINST VACCINE MANUFACTURERS?

Answer: It depends on several factors. As vaccines are the cornerstone of
global and national public health programs, many vaccine-producing countries have developed special policies to protect the vaccine supply chain.
Among those policies are vaccine injury compensation programs (VICPs).
These are often called "no-fault" programs because they provide compensation for consumers who have suffered specified types of adverse effects after
being vaccinated, while also shielding vaccine manufacturers from certain
kinds of legal liability. As of 2020, 25 countries have such programs in place.

In the United States, individuals or families that believe they have been
injured by vaccines can bring their case to the national VICP. Between
2006 and 2019, approximately 71 percent of the cases brought to the program were awarded compensation. In the same time period, over 4 billion
doses of vaccine were administered. That comes to one case of compensation for vaccine adverse effects out of every one million doses of vaccines.
Over $4 billion has been awarded in compensation since the program
started in 1988, with an average award of approximately $100,000 to pay

for health care costs. Legal fees are paid by the VICP, whether or not compensation is awarded (Thompson, 2020).

During the COVID-19 pandemic, the Secretary of Health and Human Services issued the Public Readiness and Emergency Preparedness Act (PREP Act), which limits liability for all medical countermeasures, including vaccines. That means that manufacturers of COVID-19 vaccines cannot be sued for alleged injuries, as long as they follow all applicable public health guidelines, regulations, and safety procedures.

The Facts: National vaccine compensation programs that use the no-fault model have become standard in both vaccine-producing and vaccine-importing countries, but they remain controversial among consumers. Proponents argue that vaccine manufacturers will simply leave the market if they do not have protection against unlimited lawsuits. Consumer advocates argue that it is not fair or reasonable to expect parents of an injured child, or an adult who has been injured by a vaccine, to take on a huge, complex, and expensive legal battle against Big Pharma in order to receive compensation for the injury.

Opponents of the no-fault model argue that if companies are shielded from legal liability, they may not be as active in promoting quality control. They also point out that the set of injuries for which consumers can be compensated is very limited. There is an approved list of known adverse effects for which consumers may claim compensation, and cases involving those adverse effects can be settled quickly. But if consumers claim other adverse effects, not previously documented, the cases can take much longer to settle, and compensation is much less certain.

The first country to implement VICP was Germany, in 1961. It arose out of a Supreme Court decision in 1953 to provide compensation to those who could document adverse effects from mandatory smallpox vaccination. During the 1970s, other countries began to debate similar programs, as the number of lawsuits rose involving adverse effects from the diphtheria, tetanus, and pertussis vaccine.

Within the United States, hearings on VICPs were first held in Congress in the 1980s. At that time, all the major vaccine manufacturers were based in the United States, in effect providing vaccines to the entire world. As Congressman Henry Waxman explained, "Today's hearings are an attempt to deal with the difficult problems of vaccine injury and vaccine supply. Vaccines and immunizations have worked miracles in this country. . . . But because of insurance, liability problems, and manufacturers' pricing structures, vaccines are becoming the fastest rising cost in the health economy" (Waxman, 1986).

Vaccines are in fact very hard to make. Companies that decide to invest in their research and development have to expect to make costly, long-term commitments to laboratory facilities, manufacturing plants, and government regulation. For every 15 vaccine candidates that a company may invest in, only one will make it all the way through the process of initial promise, all three phases of clinical trials, and FDA approval. Estimates of the cost of developing a single vaccine have risen from $231 million in 1991 to $1 billion in 2010. The cost of building manufacturing plants alone can cost between $50 million and $300 million.

Even beyond the cost, pharmaceutical companies face many challenges in developing vaccines. The basic biology of the organisms that cause the disease must be well established by science, and there must be some reason for thinking that an effective vaccine can be made. Also, vaccines are highly specialized. Each one has to be uniquely designed for the specific microorganism it is treating, and so the science and manufacturing knowledge required to develop one cannot be automatically applied to other diseases. This is in contrast to medications like painkillers, for example, which can be used for a wide range of diseases.

Any vaccine developed also has to have a clear pathway for testing on animals before it can be used on humans. If there aren't suitable animal subjects, there is no way to meet the regulatory requirements for clinical trials. This requirement is one of the factors that has hindered research on a vaccine against the human immunodeficiency virus (HIV).

Another challenge is the human immune system itself. It is highly adapted for protecting people against pathogens, but it is also hard for researchers to predict its response. Extensive testing using thousands of clinical subjects is necessary to ensure that any vaccine candidate is both efficacious and safe. In addition, any changes or additions to the vaccine candidates, including those projected to be improvements to the design or manufacturing process, must be clinically tested again to ensure nothing has changed with regard to its safety or efficacy.

The cost to meet all these challenges must be paid up-front, as an initial investment into the process. In financial terms, the company must assume all the initial risk. Still, the rewards can be considerable. Once a vaccine production line is well established, it may only cost between $3 and $6 per dose to produce, meaning that most of a $20–$60 price per dose is profit. And once a vaccine is part of a national or international vaccination schedule, then that profit can be relied upon, year after year.

In national emergencies like the COVID-19 pandemic, a new vaccine may not only be profitable in itself but may also lead to rising stock prices for the vaccine manufacturer. In 2021, Pfizer was reported to have generated $3.5 billion in revenue from its COVID-19 vaccine, with perhaps 20 percent of that as profit. The stock prices of all the successful COVID-19 vaccine makers went up as the vaccines became available. However, companies like CureVac, whose vaccine candidates failed early clinical trials, saw their stock prices fall as much as 50 percent.

Through the 1980s, adding to these risks was the risk of being sued. To deal with this risk, vaccine manufacturers, like other companies, purchase liability insurance. If they are sued, then the insurance helps pay the legal costs. However, in the 1980s, as the number of lawsuits went above the limits set by insurance, the cost of liability insurance increased. Just as people whose car insurance suddenly increases may have second thoughts about whether they can afford to drive, so too companies that had been manufacturing vaccines had second thoughts about the risks of producing vaccines versus the rewards. As the risk of being hit with expensive lawsuits increased, a number of companies stopped producing vaccines. This, in turn, led to vaccine shortages that left children more vulnerable to vaccine-preventable diseases.

In the hearings, Waxman argued that the proliferation of lawsuits was not helping consumers, either. Lawsuits were expensive and time-consuming, and their outcomes were uncertain. Despite a few high-profile successes, most families found that cases involving vaccine injuries were hard to win or settle. Parents might spend years in court and end up with little or no compensation. As Waxman said, "I believe that most parents who sue manufacturers are doing so because they have a sick or injured child who needs care. Those parents now have only the court system to turn to for help, and the court system is an inefficient alternative to direct compensation."

Waxman concluded, "We cannot afford to price vaccines out of the market or let injured children go unattended. Either result will end the success of the immunization program" (Waxman, 1986). The result of these and other hearings was the national VICP, established in 1988 and amended in 2016. It has two purposes. The first is to "ensure that individuals injured by certain vaccines are provided with fair and efficient compensation." The second is to "ensure a stable vaccine supply by limiting liability for vaccine manufacturers and vaccine administrators" (HRSA).

The program pays legal fees, whether the petition for compensation is successful or not. That lifts the burden off of families, who in a civil lawsuit would have to pay for their own lawyers if they lost the case. Funding for the VICP comes from an excise tax of $.75 per dose of vaccine.

Waxman realized that the act was a series of compromises. "Manufacturers would undoubtedly prefer greater insulation from liability. Parents of injured children would certainly prefer larger compensation and fewer restrictions on court activity" (Waxman, 1986). Recent surveys indicate that those attitudes are still common today.

Most vaccine compensation programs are found in high-income countries, including Canada, Germany, France, the United Kingdom, China, Korea, and Japan. Nepal and Vietnam, two countries ranked by the UN as lower- to middle-income, also have government-run VICPs.

Throughout the world, individuals who believe they or their children have been injured by the program must start the process. In the United States, that is through filing a claim with the VICP. Most claims are filed by lawyers who specialize in vaccine law. As legal expenses are paid by the program, consumers do not have to pay out of pocket. Not all lawyers handle vaccine cases, and in fact consumers indicated that finding a lawyer in their area may be difficult.

If the injury already appears on the table of vaccine injuries maintained by the program, then compensation can be awarded quickly. For example, the majority of recent cases have been for adverse effects from the seasonal influenza vaccine, including shoulder injury relating to vaccine administration. If the injury does not appear on the table, then consumers can still petition for compensation, but the process will take longer and require more documentation. The amount of time it can take for a case to work its way through the system is the most common complaint among all vaccine injury compensation programs. The VICP tries to clear all its cases within three years, but most people involved in the process consider that a very long time to wait for compensation.

The perceived benefits of the programs are that they do award fair compensation for vaccine-related injuries, and they have been successful in maintaining confidence in national immunization programs.

FURTHER READING

Douglas, R. Gordon, and Vijay B. Samant. 2018. "The Vaccine Industry." In *Plotkin's Vaccines* (Elsevier): 41–50. https://www.ncbi.nlm.nih.gov/pmc/articles/PMC7151793/.

Holland, Mary. 2018. "Liability for Vaccine Injury: The United States, the European Union, and the Developing World." *Emory Law Journal* 67: 415–62. https://scholarlycommons.law.emory.edu/elj/vol67/iss3/3.

Mungwira, Randy, Christine Guillard, Adiela Saldaña, Nobuhiko Okabe, Helen Petousis-Harris, Edinam Agbenu, Lance Rodewald, and Patrick Zuber. 2020. "Global Landscape Analysis of No-Fault Compensation

Programmes for Vaccine Injuries: A Review and Survey of Implementing Countries." *PLoS One*: 21. https://journals.plos.org/plosone /article?id=10.1371/journal.pone.0233334.

"The PREP Act and COVID-19: Limiting Liability for Medical Countermeasures." 2021. *Congressional Research Office*. https://crsreports.congress .gov/product/pdf/LSB/LSB10443.

Thompson, Kimberly, Walter Orenstein, and Alan Hinman. 2020. "Performance of the United States Vaccine Injury Compensation Program (VICP): 1988–2019." *Vaccine* 38 (9): 2136–43. https://doi.org/10.1016 /j.vaccine.2020.01.042.

U.S. Department of Health Resources and Services Administration (HRSA). n.d. "National Vaccination Injury Compensation Program." Accessed February 23, 2022. https://www.hrsa.gov/vaccine-compensation /index.html.

U.S. Government Accountability Office. 2014. "Vaccine Injury Compensation. Most Claims Took Multiple Years and Many Were Settled through Negotiation." GAO-15-142, November 21, 2014. https://www.gao .gov/products/gao-15-142.

Waxman, Henry. 1986. In *Vaccine Injury Compensation. Hearing before the Subcommittee on Health and the Environment of the Committee on Energy and Commerce. United States House of Representatives.* 99th Congress, 2nd session, July 25, 1986.

World Health Organization (WHO). n.d. "Vaccines and Immunization." Accessed August 17, 2021. https://www.who.int/health-topics/vaccines -and-immunization-tab=tab_1.

5

❖

Vaccines for a Healthier Future

INTRODUCTION

As we begin to come to grips with the implications of the COVID-19 pandemic, one of the key questions has to be, Where do we go from here? In this section, we will explore some of the ways that vaccine scientists, public health agencies, governments, philanthropic organizations, and individuals are applying lessons learned to build a healthier future. What organizations are working on expanding vaccine development and access, and what are their strategic plans? What steps can we take to maintain ongoing research on vaccines against known infectious diseases, and how can we protect ourselves against those that are previously unknown, like COVID-19? How can we protect vaccine supply chains against shortages, disruptions, crime, and fraud? How can we improve vaccine confidence, so that more people who have access to vaccines will agree to take them? And how can we apply what we learned to help prevent future sickness and death from vaccine-preventable disease?

As we look back at the 20 years preceding the pandemic, we can see how many warnings we received about our potential vulnerability. Emerging human coronaviruses had been close to the top of the list of pathogens of concern highlighted by the World Health Organization and other international public health agencies ever since the SARS and MERS epidemics. The Coalition for Epidemic Preparedness and Innovation had been launched in 2017 specifically to fund data collection and other research into vaccines capable of defending against emerging infectious diseases. Science writer David Quammen's award-winning book, *Spillover*, described in detail exactly how diseases jumped from animal to human hosts and how quickly they could spread along modern transportation networks. Popular movies from *Outbreak* (1995) to *Contagion* (2011) portrayed, dramatically and convincingly, how outbreaks could become epidemics and then pandemics. Even the video game *Plague Inc.* (released in 2012) was based on real-world, plausible assumptions about how deadly disease could spread around the world.

And yet, when the real thing happened, country after country, public health agency after public health agency, and community after community were caught unprepared. Some of the reasons for the unpreparedness are clear in hindsight. Many of the world's vaccine-have countries and regions had become complacent. It had been so long since they had experienced a serious health care crisis that they no longer thought of infectious disease as a threat. Public health budgets had been pared down to pay for other types of social services. Vaccine research was underfunded compared to other medical science specialties. At the same time, many health care systems in vaccine-have-not countries and regions faced many basic challenges. Existing funding was already stretched to capacity, and resources for dealing with the pandemic were dependent on international public health agencies.

Another factor was that although scientists can quickly map the genetic code for new pathogens, they cannot predict—or prevent—the ways mutations allow microorganisms to turn human environments to their own advantage. Once COVID-19 reached outbreak status, all the foresight in the world couldn't have contained it to a single city or a single country. Our world is too interconnected for that.

And so preventing future global pandemics requires global strategic planning. Key to that planning is understanding as much as possible about infectious diseases and how they can be contained, from the time a pathogen emerges to the last dose of vaccine given to the last vulnerable individual. Tools of modern science allow us to identify likely pathogens and to research and develop vaccine candidates more quickly than ever before. We can also study supply chains and plan in advance for transportation networks and storage units placed strategically throughout the world. We can plan for quality assurance and security measures to keep vaccine research, manufacturing, and distribution safe from crime and corruption. We can build on and improve global funding mechanisms for ensuring that lower- to middle-income countries have the same equitable access to vaccines as high-income countries. We can do more to incorporate childhood, young adult, and adult vaccine schedules into resilient health care infrastructure around the world, so that all 27 currently available vaccines are truly accessible to all.

In addition, we can find new ways to build confidence in the power of vaccines to genuinely prevent and eliminate vaccine-preventable diseases. If the pandemic taught us many sobering lessons, it also taught us how resilient we can be, even in the face of the worst health care crisis many of us have known. We can build on that resilience to provide more, and more accessible, vaccines for a healthier future.

Q33. IS IT POSSIBLE TO INCREASE VACCINATION WORLDWIDE AND DECREASE THE RISK OF VACCINE-PREVENTABLE DISEASES?

Answer: Yes. National and international public health agencies have developed strategic plans to increase and improve vaccination rates worldwide and decrease the risk of vaccine-preventable disease outbreaks. Internationally, the two most influential agencies are the World Health Organization (WHO) and the United Nations Children's Fund (UNICEF). The strategic plans established by the United States Centers for Disease Control and Prevention (CDC) are also highly influential, as the United States is a major vaccine-producing country as well as a major supporter of global health care initiatives. GAVI, the Vaccine Alliance, has also developed strategic plans as part of its mission to provide vaccines to the world's poorest countries.

Until the end of the 19th century, the only available vaccine was for smallpox. Planning was left up to individual initiatives and market forces. Individual doctors ordered the supplies they needed for their patients, and individual vaccine companies manufactured the vaccine based on their expected orders. In wartime, governments often contracted with manufacturers to deliver doses in bulk, and civilian governments tried to do the same during outbreaks. The process was very cumbersome, with many delays and shortages.

During the early 20th century, vaccine availability increased, and public health planning improved. Some countries and regions instituted mandatory vaccines for smallpox and other diseases, which were often administered in school. As the number of schoolchildren each year could be estimated to a high degree of accuracy, public health officials and vaccine manufacturers could plan ahead. This reduced delays and shortages and made for more effective vaccination programs.

In the second half of the 20th century, many factors drove continued growth in vaccination programs, both nationally and worldwide. More vaccines were developed for people and animals than ever before, and both national agencies and WHO regulated them to ensure they were safe and effective. Once the vaccines were established as being essential for the health and well-being of children and adults, WHO and UNICEF made it a priority to make them accessible to children in poor countries. That meant considerable logistical planning to get vaccines from the wealthy countries where they were made to poor countries where they were desperately needed.

In the 21st century, national and international plans for distributing vaccinations to all populations faced a number of challenges, including funding limits, transportation difficulties, and inequitable access. If production and sales of vaccines are left to market forces, what happens to poorer people in wealthy countries, or poorer countries throughout the world? If vaccine cold storage requires constant electricity, then how can vaccines be distributed to places far off the electric grid? To overcome these challenges, vaccination strategic plans had to be revised and tailored to the daily lives of their intended recipients.

Of course, even the best-laid plans can be disrupted by emergencies. The COVID-19 pandemic acted as a major disruptor, revealing all the gaps and shortcomings of previous planning documents. Previous 21st-century outbreaks, such as severe acute respiratory syndrome (SARS, 2003), Middle East respiratory syndrome (MERS, 2012), and Ebola (2014–16), had been the kind of warning shot that led some public health officials to plan for future epidemics. But the consensus among global public health experts was that too many national and international agencies had ignored those warnings.

In the future, a key component of any vaccination strategic plan will be to avoid complacency. Vaccine-preventable diseases are still very much in circulation and continue to threaten the world's human and animal population. As COVID-19 has shown, the question is not if there will be another pandemic, but when. Effective public health strategic planning can help make the next pandemic less deadly and destructive.

The Facts: Many organizations have a strategic planning process to help guide decision-making. A strategic plan sets priorities for the organization that align with the organization's mission. The plan sets out goals to be achieved, often within a specific timeframe, as well as the concrete steps to be taken to achieve the goals. A large organization may have an overall strategic plan, with each department developing its own plan, aligned with the organization's goals but tailored to the activities of that department.

A key component of a strategic plan is communication. An effective plan should convey the organization's priorities to other people within the organization as well as to external stakeholders. Stakeholders can be anyone who has a stake in the organization's success, including clients or customers, partners, investors, and government bodies.

Other key components are accountability and assessment. An effective strategic plan should communicate what departments or individuals will be held accountable for carrying out specific tasks. It should also establish how it will assess how well those tasks have been carried out.

WHO's *Immunization Agenda 2030* provides a road map for immunization programs within its larger role in promoting global health. Its vision is "a world where everyone, everywhere, at every age, fully benefits from vaccines for good health and well-being." This vision statement can be directly tied to three strategic goals. WHO regional offices and national and local partners can then focus on the concrete steps that must be completed by 2030 to achieve those goals—including the overarching goal of reducing "mortality and morbidity from vaccine-preventable diseases for everyone throughout the life course." This, in turn, can be directly related to more targeted goals, such as increasing the number of vaccinated children worldwide, the number of adolescent girls who receive the human papillomavirus (HPV) vaccine, and the number of adults who receive influenza and COVID-19 vaccines. As the report notes, increased rates of vaccination between 2010 and 2017 cut the mortality rate of children under age five around the world by 24 percent; the introduction of the HPV vaccine led to a 51 percent decrease in precancerous lesions in girls ages 15–19.

WHO's goal to "leave no one behind, by increasing equitable access and use of new and existing vaccines" is a daunting one. People who live in wealthy countries have easy access to all approved vaccines, but millions of people in poor or conflict-ridden countries struggle to get routine vaccines like those for diphtheria, tetanus, and pertussis (DPT) or measles. The COVID-19 vaccine rollout underscored long-standing inequities between vaccine-have and vaccine-have-not nations. Wealthy countries stockpiled more than enough doses for all their residents, whereas poor countries struggled to obtain enough doses just to vaccinate frontline health care workers.

WHO has long maintained that access to health care is a human right and that good health and well-being is the basis for flourishing economic and political systems. As studies have shown, vaccination programs in developing countries play a significant role in reducing burdensome health care costs and poverty overall. By 2030, economists forecast that vaccines will keep an estimated 24 million people above the global poverty line (WHO, 2020).

Whereas WHO's strategic planning stays primarily at the policy level, UNICEF's *Immunization Roadmap, 2018–2030* focuses more on operations and logistics. The organization's overall mission is to ensure that "the right of every woman and every child to immunization is fully realized, with priority given to the most disadvantaged." UNICEF works with 130 countries, and the vaccines it procures reach nearly half the world's children. For the future, UNICEF, like WHO, will be focusing more on vaccination throughout the life course, so that adults as well as children can be protected against vaccine-preventable diseases (UNICEF, 2018).

UNICEF's road map notes expected advances in the next decade, such as new and improved vaccines, new storage and transportation facilities, and new delivery technologies. These come with challenges to the population UNICEF serves. In many parts of the world, economic pressures are pushing rural families into cities with overburdened health care systems and services. Basic health care, including vaccination, may be almost as inaccessible as it was when the families lived in remote rural areas. The difficulties of vaccinating children or adults in fragile or conflict-affected areas are expected to continue. And, of course, new disease threats such as COVID-19 are an ever-present concern.

Some of UNICEF's specific goals lay out precise ways to deal with vaccination coverage gaps. For areas that are geographically remote, these might involve situating vaccine administration centers at transit hubs or using coast guards to deliver them to families on remote islands. In urban settings, efforts might include mapping parts of the city with large under-vaccinated populations, providing evening or weekend hours for vaccination clinics, and using mobile technology to track shifting urban populations.

Other goals have to do with the logistics of procuring vaccines for half of the world's children. This gives UNICEF enormous purchasing power, which it can use to buy vaccines in bulk at more affordable prices. This purchasing power can also be used to encourage vaccine manufacturers to plan for sustainable delivery throughout the world, not just in wealthy countries. UNICEF's operations team can build on their experience to strengthen supply chains and transportation networks, so that vaccines can reach more families.

The CDC's focus is primarily on U.S. public health, but because both U.S. citizens and diseases have worldwide influence, their strategic planning is global in scope. The CDC's mission "is to protect the safety, health, and security of America from threats within the country's borders and around the world." The safety and security of the world contribute to the

United States' safety and security. Vaccination, both within the country and internationally, is therefore one of its priorities, as this "is among the most cost-effective ways to support a healthier and safer world." As the COVID-19 pandemic and the vaccine development process showed, vaccination programs "save lives, prevent disability, and protect livelihoods for Americans" as well as "populations around the globe" (CDC, 2021).

The CDC's *Global Immunization Strategic Framework 2021–2030* sets out five goals. The first is to *Prevent* outbreaks of vaccine-preventable diseases by building on and expanding vaccination programs. The second is to *Detect* outbreaks by maintaining strong, effective surveillance systems. The third, *Respond*, builds on the first two and includes preparation to ensure that national and global health care systems can meet the challenge of well-known as well as novel disease outbreaks. The fourth, *Sustain*, is designed to ensure that vaccination programs can be kept running continuously, that they are not put in place during outbreaks and then allowed to lapse. And the fifth, *Innovate*, ensures that scientific research into new vaccines is also ongoing, so that more and more deadly infectious diseases can become vaccine preventable.

Gavi, the Vaccine Alliance, has a very concentrated planning strategy, measured in five-year cycles rather than in decades. In "Gavi 5.0," the organization's strategic plan for 2021–25, Gavi focuses on the estimated 20 million "zero-dose" children worldwide. Zero-dose children, usually from the world's poorest and most fragile areas, are those who have received no vaccines at all—or any other kind of routine medical care. Another priority is to help poorer countries develop the kind of public health surveillance and stockpiling programs common in wealthy countries, so that they, too, can be prepared for future outbreaks.

In public health, strategic planning is essential to help prepare for and respond to otherwise unpredictable disease events like outbreaks and pandemics. Resilient, sustainable, safe, and effective vaccination programs, carefully planned and carefully executed, are our best defense against disruptions caused by vaccine-preventable diseases.

FURTHER READING

Centers for Disease Control and Prevention (CDC). 2021. *Global Immunization Strategic Framework 2021–2030*. https://www.cdc.gov/globalhealth/immunization/framework/index.html.

Gavi, the Vaccine Alliance. 2021. *Phase V (2021–2025)*. https://www.gavi.org/our-alliance/strategy/phase-5-2021-2025.

United Nations Children's Fund (UNICEF). 2018. *UNICEF Immunization Roadmap, 2018–2030.* https://www.unicef.org/sites/default/files/2019-01/UNICEF_Immunization_Roadmap_2018.pdf.

World Health Organization (WHO). 2020. *Immunization Agenda 2030: A Global Strategy to Leave No One Behind.* https://www.who.int/publications/m/item/immunization-agenda-2030-a-global-strategy-to-leave-no-one-behind.

Q34. CAN WE PREPARE IN ADVANCE TO PROVIDE VACCINES FOR EMERGING INFECTIOUS DISEASES?

Answer: Yes. Ever since the Ebola outbreaks of 2013–16 in West Africa, global public health organizations have been working to develop research, manufacturing, and distribution systems that give scientists and manufacturers the capacity to develop vaccines for infectious diseases before an epidemic strikes.

In 2017, a number of organizations came together to announce the launch of the Coalition for Epidemic Preparedness Innovations (CEPI). The mission of the organization is "is to accelerate the development of vaccines against emerging infectious diseases and enable equitable access to these vaccines for people during outbreaks" (CEPI, "About Us"). Its headquarters are in Oslo, Norway, with offices in London and in Washington, DC. It works closely with the World Health Organization (WHO) and with national public health organizations, pharmaceutical companies, and regulatory agencies around the world. Funding comes from member countries, from the World Bank, and from private philanthropies such as the Bill and Melinda Gates Foundation.

The development of the Ebola vaccine in response to the 2013–16 outbreak was in many ways a turning point for vaccine manufacturing. Previous vaccines had taken as long as 10–15 years to develop, as pharmaceutical companies worked through initial scientific development, through the three phases of vaccine trials, and then the move to full manufacturing capacity. In contrast, Ebola vaccines were approved for emergency use by 2016 and received full approval by 2019. One reason they could be developed so quickly was that much of the science involved in the vaccine was well understood by the time full-scale clinical trials were underway.

But that success led to an obvious question: if an Ebola vaccine could be developed so quickly, why hadn't it been done already? Ebola had been first identified in 1976, and there were multiple outbreaks of the disease throughout the 1990s and early 2000s. Surely it would have been possible to start vaccine development much earlier?

The delay came from the finances of vaccine development rather than the science. A single vaccine can cost as much as $1 billion to develop. Each vaccine usually needs its own manufacturing system, including facility, supplies, and trained personnel, and that alone can cost around $300,000. Moreover, vaccine development is very risky: only one in 15 vaccine candidates make it to final authorization for clinical use. And once a vaccine is successfully administered, it puts itself out of business for that person. That is, that person will never need the vaccine again, unlike medications taken for chronic illness.

Many pharmaceutical companies have historically been very reluctant to tie up their resources in developing vaccines unless they have been given financial incentives, usually from governments of wealthy countries. These incentives make take the form of grants for research and manufacturing, or contracts that guarantee the number of units that will be purchased. During the COVID-19 pandemic, pharmaceutical companies that had the necessary capacity were offered both forms of incentives, which enabled them to produce the vaccines in under a year.

The difficulty in applying that model to Ebola, as well as other diseases like Zika and Lassa fever, is that they primarily affect a limited number of people in developing nations. There has historically been little financial incentive for pharmaceutical companies to devote resources to developing vaccines. The countries affected by these diseases do not have the financial resources available to wealthy nations to purchase expensive vaccines. Neither do they have the scientific or manufacturing or economic capacity to develop vaccines within their own borders.

The idea behind CEPI is to harness public and private donors to provide funding for vaccine research and distribution. From 2022 through 2026, the organization plans to raise $3.5 billion to be spend on all aspects of the vaccine development process, from discovery, through development and licensure, to manufacture, delivery and/or stockpiling, to the "last mile": administration to patients.

The COVID-19 pandemic has underlined the urgency of advance planning for vaccine research and delivery. Many more national and global public health agencies have classified emerging infectious diseases as a security threat. They therefore have been devoting additional resources to ensuring that vaccines and vaccine candidates are available and ready to prevent future epidemics.

The Facts: When CEPI was launched in 2017, its targets were defined as emerging infectious diseases (EIDs), which had the potential for becoming epidemics. These had already been identified by WHO as priority diseases. Vaccine candidates for many EIDs had been tested on animals at that point, but had not progressed to human trials. These included vaccine candidates for the Nipah virus, first identified in 1999 in an outbreak among pig farmers in Malaysia. It has since been found to be endemic in a number of animal species in Asia that come into close contact with humans. When it spreads to people, it can cause severe respiratory illness and death. CEPI also supported research into vaccine candidates for Middle East respiratory syndrome (MERS), and for Lassa fever, an acute viral illness, endemic in rats, that had led to outbreaks of severe disease in West Africa. Two additional mosquito-borne diseases were later added to CEPI's list, Rift Valley fever and Chikungunya. CEPI also supports ongoing research into additional Ebola vaccine candidates.

Virologists had pointed out the dangers of animal-borne diseases for many years. They warned that any of these diseases, once they made the jump to humans, could easily lead to epidemics or even pandemics. The problem is that the cost of creating vaccines for these kinds of diseases is considerable. Human trials are costly to design, implement, and monitor. The research must be carried out where the disease is endemic, so that the infection rate of vaccinated people can be measured against that of unvaccinated people. For a disease that ordinarily has a limited geographical area, clinical trials may involve building modern research and manufacturing facilities from the ground up. They also involve working closely with government officials, and with local populations, to make sure that the research is supported by those whom it is designed to help.

By 2018, WHO had added a new category to its priority diseases, "Disease X." This was defined as an unknown infectious disease that could develop into a serious international public health crisis. As CEPI scientists noted, "By their very nature, we cannot predict what or where 'Disease X' is likely to emerge" (CEPI, "Priority Diseases"). When COVID-19 was first identified at the end of 2018, it had many of the characteristics that CEPI and WHO experts had expected: an acute viral disease that spread around the world in a matter of months. Fortunately, as a coronavirus, its molecular structure was well understood. CEPI's own prior research into MERS, as well as that of many other scientists around the world, could be harnessed in developing a vaccine. As the COVID-19 pandemic unfolded, CEPI worked with GAVI (the Vaccine Alliance) and WHO to provide funding and strategic support for COVAX, the special initiative to provide COVID-19 vaccines to low- and middle-income nations.

The COVID-19 epidemic led CEPI and other national and international organizations to reassess what could be done to protect the world's population against future pandemics. In their 2022–26 working document, CEPI officials noted that it had taken 314 days—less than a year—to develop the first vaccine against COVID-19 with Emergency Use Authorization (EUA) from the United States and WHO. Although this was a phenomenal achievement, they believed that it could and should have been done in 100 days. Taking up this challenge, the Pandemics Preparedness Partnership wrote, "Imagine a scenario where COVID-19 had hit, but the world was ready." In this scenario, within 100 days of the first case reported in Wuhan, China, in December, 2019—by May 2020, in other words—the outbreak would have been under control. Millions of lives would have been saved, lockdowns would have been shortened, and trillions of dollars in lost economic output could have been avoided.

Such a response, though, would require the same kind of serious, sustained, long-range planning that characterizes national responses to many security threats. It would start with an international surveillance system that quickly reported an unusual "flu" in Wuhan, with scientists on staff who could sequence and share the genomic data even more quickly than the 20 days it took in 2020. Existing diagnostic tests and a system of contact tracing could have been activated by public health authorities previously trained in the logistics of infectious diseases. Vaccine prototypes could already have been in the pipeline for coronaviruses, with manufacturing capacity already built and ready to be scaled up for global use. WHO would already have global standards in place for international regulatory approvals, and UNICEF and other international aid organizations would already have supply chains up and running for rapid distribution to communities at risk. And all nations could already have an agreed-upon plan for equitable distribution for vaccines and other necessary medical treatment worldwide (G7 Summit, 2021).

For the next steps against COVID-19, CEPI and its partners are putting their support toward developing vaccines that are targeted toward lower- to middle-income countries. That means redefining the idea of "efficacy" in vaccines to mean not just "effective against the pathogen" but also "designed to be distributed in the most effective way." That, in turn, means vaccines that can be delivered in a single dose so as to keep production, storage, and transportation costs down. Vaccines, to be most effective, should also provide long-lasting protection, as scheduling booster shots often is a major challenge for nations with fragile economies and the communities who live in them. Ideally, vaccines would also only require standard refrigeration for storage, rather than the special storage facilities necessary for the first set of COVID-19 vaccines.

COVID-19 is not the only coronavirus that threatens the world's population, and there are many other virus families that could lead to pandemics, under the right—or, from the human standpoint, the worst—conditions. As it is impossible to know in advance which virus outbreak might lead to an epidemic, CEPI and other organizations are supporting research into designing types of vaccines that can be adapted to specific viruses. For example, the spike protein is a well-researched aspect of coronavirus. Using mRNA technology developed for the COVID-19 vaccines, scientists are working to design a general-purpose vaccine that mimics that spike protein and can be tested through Phase 1 clinical trials. Then, when a new coronavirus is detected, the general-purpose vaccine could be adapted to its specific molecular structure. This would allow national and international public health agencies to create "libraries" of vaccine candidates, each adapted to the major virus families.

An important focus for all future vaccine research is to get more vaccines to more people in lower- to middle-income nations. This involves creating the kind of infrastructure that would allow vaccine research and development to take place throughout the world, not just in high-income countries. University systems in lower- to middle-income countries have to be strengthened, so that their own citizens can have the opportunity to be vaccine scientists. There has to be public and private investment in pharmaceutical companies, vaccine research, and manufacturing facilities in nations that are currently vaccine have-nots. Health care infrastructure and public health surveillance systems have to be strengthened, especially in the fragile communities where diseases like Ebola and Lassa fever are likely to occur. And for all this to happen, representatives from lower- and middle-income countries must be fully integrated into government boards of organizations like CEPI and other international health care agencies.

It is likely that the next decade will see more infectious diseases emerge. With investment in vaccine research and distribution, global efforts can make it possible to bring them under control in 100 days.

FURTHER READING

CEPI (Coalition for Epidemic Preparedness Innovations). n.d. "About Us." Accessed September 9, 2021. https://cepi.net/about/whoweare/.

CEPI. n.d. "New Vaccines for a Safer World." Accessed September 9, 2021. https://cepi.net/.

CEPI. n.d. "Priority Diseases." Accessed September 9, 2021. https://cepi.net/research_dev/priority-diseases/.

CEPI. n.d. *The Urgency of Now. CEPI's $3.5 billion plan to turn the tide against epidemic and pandemic infectious diseases.* Accessed September 9, 2021. https://endpandemics.cepi.net/.

G7 Summit. 2021. *100 Days Mission to Respond to Future Pandemic Threats.*
   https://assets.publishing.service.gov.uk/government/uploads/system
   /uploads/attachment_data/file/992762/100_Days_Mission_to_respond
   _to_future_pandemic_threats__3_.pdf.

Q35. CAN WE BETTER PROTECT HEALTH CARE PERSONNEL, FACILITIES, AND VACCINE SUPPLY CHAINS DURING PANDEMIC CONDITIONS?

Answer: Yes. As COVID-19 has shown, developing a vaccine may start with scientific research, but getting vaccine doses to the people who need them requires secure health care workers, facilities, and supply chains. That means protecting health care personnel, hospitals, pharmacies, and clinics from attacks or other disruptions so they can go about their business of administering vaccines to communities who need them. It also means protecting every aspect of the vaccine supply chain—including development, manufacturing, and distribution—from cyberattacks, fraud, and other criminal behavior.

Attacks on health care personnel and facilities are violations of international humanitarian law, but unfortunately, they still occur. Organizations such as Safeguarding Health in Conflict Coalition, a group of nongovernmental organizations, work to document incidents of conflict and raise awareness of the destructive nature of the attacks. Where feasible, it works with local groups to empower them to call upon local and national governments to provide protection for health care workers and medical facilities. The World Health Organization (WHO) maintains a Surveillance System for Attacks on Health Care to document violence, especially in fragile and conflict-affected regions. Health Care in Danger, an initiative of the International Committee of the Red Cross and Red Crescent (Red Cross), has an ongoing multiyear program to educate armed forces in conflict-ridden areas about the value of protecting health care services from threats and violence.

Vaccine manufacturing and development has many moving parts, and they are all organized via online pathways that include email, encoded messages, and data stored in cloud-based applications. This makes them vulnerable to cybersecurity threats. Even before COVID-19, health care organizations had seen a wave of cyberattacks. These ranged from attempts to steal classified patient data to ransomware that shut down computer-based diagnostic and treatment equipment. During the pandemic, cybersecurity experts provided advice to many of the vaccine developers on how to protect their research and manufacturing efforts from bad actors. A special task force of the United States' Cybersecurity and Infrastructure Security Agency (CISA) was tasked with ensuring that the vaccine rollout overall was protected against online hackers, disrupters, and thieves.

The need for vigilance doesn't end once the vaccine doses are packaged into vials. They still have to be transported to local sites for distribution to communities. Fraud and theft can take place at the country, regional, or local level. Vaccine supplies can be removed from the regular supply chain to be distributed to high-ranking political figures, and organized crime rings can hijack trucks carrying supplies. Any time there are shortages, bad actors may also attempt to sell fake vaccines and other medical materials through local, legitimate suppliers.

To counteract these threats, WHO has implemented the Effective Vaccine Monitoring (EVM) initiative. This sets the standard for good practice within the vaccine supply chain and provides for local monitors, who can visit health care facilities and provide a standard assessment. It helps local health care workers who dispense vaccines, including doctors, nurses, pharmacists, and specially trained vaccinators, to learn about what proper equipment and supplies should look like. In recent cases of vaccine fraud, authorities were alerted to the problem because local health care personnel noticed that there was something wrong with vaccine packaging. They were quickly able to tell that the alleged vaccines were fakes and make sure that they were not given to patients.

The Facts: It can be a long journey for vaccines from manufacturing plants to patients all over the world. National and international public health and security teams have scrutinized the process from start to finish in order to find and strengthen weak points that might otherwise prevent vaccines from getting to people and communities who need them.

One of the most difficult problems to solve has been getting the vaccines to communities in fragile and conflict-affected areas. Attacks by state actors—that is, military forces—may destroy hospitals and kill health care personnel as collateral damage. Armed, nonstate actors—gang members, organized criminal groups, or private individuals with guns—may target health care facilities in order to get access to drugs, or in order to steal and sell medical supplies. Attacks on doctor's offices, clinics, and hospitals may occur as part of a larger attack on a community or district. In some cases, health care personnel and facilities may even become direct targets because of vaccination efforts, if misinformation spreads that they are responsible for the disease, or if the vaccine causes side effects.

Starting in 2019, WHO set up a special international effort, the Surveillance System for Attacks on Health Care, to track and accurately report cases of violence against health care workers. Prior to that, although everyone was aware that incidents occurred, they could be hard to document. During periods of armed conflict, it was often hard to have any kind of accountability. Accounts of attacks on health care personnel or other civilians were often dismissed as propaganda.

WHO's Surveillance System includes mechanisms for verifying accounts of violence and standardizing information. It tracks violence that affects patients, personnel, facilities, and transportation. It also tracks the type of attack, such as whether it involves individual weapons, psychological violence such as threats and intimidation, heavy weapons, and outright assault. In the first nine months of 2021, WHO recorded 665 attacks in 14 countries and territories, with 210 deaths and 297 injuries.

In areas where violence is caused by unstable and vulnerable living conditions rather than armed political conflict, human rights organizations have been working to educate weapon-bearing groups about the value of protecting health care personnel and facilities from targeted or random violent crime. As part of the Health Care in Danger movement, Red Cross staff work with health care staff and with armed groups responsible for violence, whether those groups are affiliated with the state or not. They have successfully brokered agreements to protect health care workers and facilities among rival armed factions. As one of their public service advertising campaigns proclaims: "Attacks on health care providers endanger us all. Violence again health care must end. It's a matter of life and death."

Cybersecurity experts work to protect vaccine development, manufacturing, and supply chains against other kinds of attacks, involving theft of confidential data and processes and ransomware attacks on health care facilities and research laboratories. Early in the process of COVID-19 vaccine development, one group sent spoofing emails, purporting to be from a major supplier, in order to gain access to credentials that would allow them access to privileged, high-level information. Cybersecurity experts warned pharmaceutical companies that they would have to adopt a "zero-trust approach" and operate under the assumption that no part of their processes were automatically trustworthy. Companies should require that every email, and every communication, be authenticated. All documents should be handled as securely as possible. And all aspects of the manufacturing and distribution process should be protected from bad actors who might seek to disrupt it.

In the United States, CISA created a special task force to monitor cybersecurity issues in protecting COVID-19 vaccines. Initially, there were

30 companies that the task force listed as high priority, but the more that the task force looked at the problem, the more they realized that many more businesses had to be part of the effort. Many large international companies, such as Pfizer and Moderna, had long been aware of the dangers of cyberattacks and had their own in-house security experts. However, there were many smaller companies that made essential ingredients for the vaccines but they never had any reason to think about cybersecurity. According to CISA advisor Josh Corman, "You could sneeze on that one company, and they would be disrupted. And if they were disrupted, we'd be living in a very different world right now because they were so critical to those mRNA candidates" (Wetsman, 2021). The CISA team reached out to all the players, major and minor, who provided necessary supplies, equipment, or services for the vaccination effort. In making it clear that they could provide expertise, they created trust and helped build partnerships. The cybersecurity protocols put in place for the COVID-19 vaccines are expected to be standard practice for new vaccine development in the future.

Cyber fraud and information theft are online versions of the fraud and theft of medical supplies that is an ongoing problem at vaccine distribution centers. The final leg of a vaccine's journey to a patient almost always involves being loaded onto a vehicle, placed in a storage facility, and transported to a clinic, pharmacy, or medical center. In the course of that process, there may well be opportunities for real vaccine supplies to be siphoned off and sold for a higher, black-market price, or for fake supplies to be introduced into supply chains and sold as the real vaccine.

A series of such cases arose in the African nation of Niger in 2015 and 2017. Outbreaks of meningitis C during those years caused unexpected demand for available meningitis vaccines, which led to a shortage of supplies. In seeking to make up the shortfall, national public health officials purchased supplies from neighboring countries. A month into the first outbreak, a health care worker noticed that the ink on the expiration date of some of the vaccine vials looked smudged. She had attended training sessions on substandard or falsified products and suspected that the vaccine supplies she'd been given might have been fake. She notified national regulators, who in turn notified the vaccine manufacturers and WHO. The manufacturers were able to tell from photographs that the vaccines were fake: the type of vial and the label were both incorrect.

During the 2017 outbreak in Niger, it became clear that purveyors of fake vaccines had gotten more skilled. The labels were much more expertly printed, and the product information on the cartons, though fake, was convincing at first glance. Just as phishing scams have improved over the years, so too has the production and distribution of fake vaccines. The best protection against these kinds of fakes is to ensure that enough supplies of genuine vaccines are available when needed.

In many cases of fake vaccines, local health care providers notice that there's something wrong and report it to national or international authorities. WHO's EVM system is designed to make the process more systematic. It is both a process and a tool. The process involves a range of people, from the EVM leader, typically a member of the country or region's highest-level public health authority, to the EVM manager, who is tasked with organizing local-level assessments. The EVM assessors are usually health care personnel with some experience in supply chain logistics. They are assigned to each health care facility, and they interview facility managers and health care workers. The tool is a questionnaire available on a variety of phone, tablet, and computer platforms. It started in 2008 as a paper questionnaire designed to collect information from facility managers and health care workers about what actually went on at their point in the supply chain. It has since evolved to a flexible information-gathering tool with room for extensive comments and uploaded images. It can be tailored to the specific needs of a country or region.

These three types of threats to vaccine supply chains—outright violence against health care, cyberattacks, and physical fraud and theft—pose many challenges. The solution to all three, while different in many ways, is similar in one respect. They all rely on trust building, education, and transparency to make sure that all those involved in the vaccine supply chain understand its importance to the health and safety of their own communities.

FURTHER READING

Columbus, Lewis. 2021. "10 Ways Covid-19 Vaccine Supply Chains Need to Be Protected by Cybersecurity." *Forbes*. https://www.forbes.com/sites/louiscolumbus/2021/01/24/10-ways-covid-19-vaccine-supply-chains-need-to-be-protected-by-cybersecurity/?sh=ce07cc626c27.

International Committee of the Red Cross and Red Crescent. n.d. *A Matter of Life and Death. Tackling violence against health care in Iraq, Lebanon and the Philippines. Selected experiences*. Accessed September 14, 2021. https://healthcareindanger.org/wp-content/uploads/2020/08/4448_002_HCID_selected_experiences_2_ICRC.pdf.

Interpol. 2020. *Global Landscape on Covid-19 Cyberthreat*. https://www.interpol.int/en/Crimes/Cybercrime/COVID-19-cyberthreats.

Safeguarding Health in Conflict Coalition. n.d. *Safeguarding Health in Conflict. Protecting Health Workers, Services, and Infrastructure.* Accessed September 10, 2021. https://www.safeguardinghealth.org/sites/shcc/files /safeguarding-health-in-conflict-overview.pdf.

Wetsman, Nicole. 2021. "The Covid-19 Vaccines Weren't Hacked—This Task Force Is One Reason Why." *The Verge.* https://www.theverge .com/2021/7/8/22568397/covid-vaccine-cybersecurity-cisa-task-force.

World Health Organization (WHO). n.d. "Effective Vaccine Management (EVM)." Accessed September 10, 2021. https://www.who.int/teams /immunization-vaccines-and-biologicals/essential-programme-on -immunization/supply-chain/effective-vaccine-management-(evm).

WHO. n.d. "Surveillance System for Attacks on Health Care (SSA)." Accessed September 10, 2021. https://extranet.who.int/ssa/Index.aspx.

WHO. 2017. *WHO Global Surveillance System for Substandard and Falsified Medical Products.* https://www.who.int/publications/i/item/9789241513425.

Q36. CAN WE BUILD HIGHER LEVELS OF CONFIDENCE IN THE SAFETY AND EFFICACY OF VACCINES?

Answer: Yes. Though vaccine hesitancy may never entirely disappear, experts believe that public health organizations and communities can take additional steps to build public confidence in vaccines.

The U.S. Department of Health and Human Services defines vaccine confidence as "the trust that parents, patients, or providers have in:

- recommended vaccines;
- providers who administer vaccines; and
- processes and policies that lead to vaccine development, licensure, manufacturing, and recommendations for use" (HHS, "Featured Priorities").

Studies have shown that worldwide, the overwhelming majority of people are vaccine confident, ranging from 70 percent to 85 percent of the population. Factors that contribute to vaccine confidence are ongoing access to high-quality, cost-effective health care throughout the life cycle, strong positive feelings toward health care providers, and confidence in the process by which governments and public health officials make decisions. People are more likely to be vaccine confident if they have had ongoing positive experiences with health care providers, so that they think of doctors, nurses, and hospitals as places they go for successful treatment of illnesses and injuries. They are more likely to be vaccine confident if they have had positive experiences with health insurance companies, so that they have not had to pay huge medical bills out of pocket. And they are more likely to be vaccine confident if they believe that national, state, and local public health authorities are taking effective, science-based measures to protect their health and that of their communities.

An additional factor that affects vaccine confidence has to do with the perception of risk associated with a particular disease. This came out particularly strongly during the COVID-19 pandemic. Younger people, who believed they were not at high risk for dangerous symptoms if they caught the disease, were more likely to express lack of trust in the vaccines themselves and in the process by which the vaccines received Emergency Use Authorization. People aged 60 and up, who were at much greater risk for hospitalization and death from the virus, were much more likely to express trust in the process and to be vaccinated.

There is also a difference in risk perception, and thus in vaccine confidence, associated with the vaccine for human papillomavirus (HPV). The vaccine is recommended for both girls and boys aged 10 through 12. As they are children, their parents or guardians must make the decision to have them vaccinated. Parents of girls are more likely to decide on vaccination, because there is a clear link between HPV and cancers of the female reproductive system, most notably cervical cancer. Although there is an equally clear link between HPV infections and penile cancer, penile cancer is rare, and it may seem like less of a risk to parents of boys. Fortunately, there is enough overall confidence in HPV vaccines to make a significant difference in public health. As the HPV vaccine was added to the list of recommended vaccines in the United States, the number of HPV infections, including precancerous cells, has decreased by 88 percent.

A key tool in increasing vaccine confidence is increasing access, which means removing barriers to high-quality, cost-effective health care. Other tools include providing clear, accurate information about vaccines, expanding opportunities for communication with communities, and encouraging research into the causes of vaccine confidence and vaccine hesitancy.

The Facts: Public health discussions of vaccine confidence in the United States predated the COVID-19 pandemic. In 2014–15, cases of measles brought to the United States by families who had traveled abroad led to a set of outbreaks, particularly associated with Disneyland Resorts in Anaheim, California. Measles was widely perceived as being eliminated in the United States, and so the outbreak received widespread attention from public health authorities and from news media. It became clear that children who developed measles had not been vaccinated, even though the vaccine had been available to their families. This, in turn, spurred new research as to why some families were vaccine confident while others were vaccine hesitant.

In 2015, the National Vaccine Advisory Committee, under the U.S. Department of Health and Human Services (HSS), commissioned a working group to report on the state of vaccine confidence in the United States, particularly with respect to the recommended childhood vaccination schedule. The working group determined that there are four factors that were especially important in vaccine confidence. The first is trust, particularly trust in "someone else's expertise and advice (e.g., their vaccine recommendation)." For vaccines, this means not just trust in a primary health care provider—for example, a pediatrician—but also trust in pharmaceutical companies, regulatory bodies, and public health authorities.

A second factor is "attitudes and beliefs" parents may have regarding "vaccine safety, vaccine effectiveness, and vaccination benefits." They are more likely to have confidence in vaccines if they perceive the vaccine-preventable disease is something their children are likely to encounter, if they perceive it poses a serious threat to their children, and if they perceive the vaccine as safe. One underlying cause of the measles outbreak was that some parents perceived measles as a disease that had already been eliminated and thus was unlikely to affect their children. They also thought of it as a mild disease that could do no permanent damage.

Other factors had to do with the information environment in which parents existed. Parental attitudes are greatly affected by the norms and beliefs of the social groups to which they belong, as well as their preferred news sources. If many parents in their social circle were vaccinated, and they paid attention to news outlets that released accurate information about vaccines and public health, parents were much more likely to be supportive of vaccination for themselves and their children. In effect, the social norms fostered a vaccine confidence support network.

Of course, this could work the other way as well. Already by 2015, the vaccine confidence working group noted phenomena that would become significant during the COVID-19 pandemic: the tendency of vaccine-hesitant individuals and communities to follow news and social media that reinforced their hesitancy. As the report noted, "Social media platforms can become virtual echo chambers for fostering questions about vaccine safety and can reinforce false information and myths" ("Assessing the State of Vaccine Confidence," 2015).

Based on its research, the vaccine confidence working group made a number of recommendations. One was to work with state and local public health authorities to put in place a system to collect more data, specifically on factors that affected vaccine confidence. This would address the fact that data based on national or even state-level vaccination rates might mask local variations. They also recommended collecting data that looked more closely at issues of trust, of attitudes and beliefs, and of information environments, in addition to vaccination rates. They recommended working with primary health care providers, especially pediatricians, to encourage trust-building practices and to counter misinformation.

All these recommendations were put into effect during a 2017 measles outbreak in Hennepin County, Minnesota. There are approximately 1.2 million residents in the county, with a 89 percent measles, mumps, rubella (MMR) vaccination rate overall. However, approximately 13 percent of the county's population were Somali-American, and their vaccination rate was initially only 42 percent. As a result, when a measles outbreak occurred in the county, most of the children affected were Somali-Minnesotan. About 9,000 individuals were exposed, with 70 confirmed cases and 22 hospitalizations.

Hennepin County public health officials took active steps to encourage families to vaccinate their children. They contacted primary health care providers, asking them to check their records and contact parents whose children had not received the recommended MMR vaccine. They worked with trusted community leaders, who made over 150 visits to apartments, workplaces, community centers, and mosques to share information and dispel myths about vaccination. They made home visits to families who did not own phones or who could not be reached in other settings. The visits from trusted individuals "particularly helped with reluctant individuals and provided a comfortable setting for candid discussions about their reluctance." The number of vaccinations increased from approximately 200 within the Somali-Minnesotan community to 1,600 (National Vaccine Program Office, 2017).

Similar case studies have shown the value of trusted community leaders and primary health care providers in increasing vaccine confidence. However, what if individuals and families don't seek out such information but instead look to online sources when deciding about vaccination? During the COVID-19 pandemic, many observers noted that online misinformation, disinformation, and outright fraud played a significant role in reducing vaccine confidence.

In his 2021 report, *Confronting Health Misinformation: The U.S. Surgeon General's Advisory on Building a Healthy Information Environment*, Attorney General Dr. Vivek Murthy called on journalists, media organizations, and technology organizations to take a much more active role in creating a supportive information environment for vaccination programs and for health information overall. The report called on journalists and media organizations to be trained in identifying misinformation and to treat it as inaccurate and misleading in their reporting. It urged journalists to embrace their role in keeping the public informed. Murthy also called on news organizations to choose headlines and images that provide clear information about health care, rather than choosing content for the purpose of trying to shock or provoke their audiences. It further recommended that journalists report local, community-based stories, which would encourage trust between communities and public health authorities.

The report's most pointed criticisms were aimed at technology companies such as Facebook, YouTube, and Twitter, which were widely blamed for spreading misinformation that hindered COVID-19 public health efforts. The report urged companies to take seriously the harms that their hands-off policy had done in allowing the spread of misinformation and to "take responsibility for addressing the harms." Specific recommendations made to social media companies included greater investment in the monitoring and removal of misinformation. The report also urged these companies to adjust their algorithms to avoid recommending posts with misinformation.

The report claimed that social media companies needed to make other changes as well. They should build in "frictions—such as suggestions and warnings," which have been shown reduce the sharing of misinformation online. They should take steps to identify "superspreaders" of misinformation and impose clear penalties for repeat offenders. Where there are information deficits—areas where lack of certainty can lead to myths and half-truths—technology companies should adjust their algorithms to provide links to trusted, science-based sources. Communications from trusted, accurate sources should be amplified, so it is not drowned out by waves of misinformation—and people who provide trusted, accurate information should be protected from online harassment. Above all, technology companies need to be transparent about their data and provide it to legitimate researchers to allow them to learn more about the range and impact of health care misinformation (HSS, 2021). The main technology platforms have acknowledged their responsibility to look for ways to build confidence in legitimate health care information, including information about vaccination.

The National Science Foundation (NSF), which funds research in the sciences, has provided a series of grants on "Trust and Authenticity in Communications." Since communication is at the core of much of modern civic, economic, and scientific life, there is a tremendous need for research on how to strengthen production and distribution of accurate, trustworthy communication, and prevent the proliferation of misinformation, disinformation, and fraud. 2021 awardees include teams at MIT, to develop a software tool to address vaccine hesitancy and misinformation, the University of Washington, to develop educational programs to promote digital literacy in historically underserved populations, and George Washington University, to investigate the connection between misinformation communities and online harassment campaigns.

As the COVID-19 pandemic made clear, vaccine confidence cannot be taken for granted. Public health authorities, communication specialists, and scientific experts have all made it a priority as an essential feature of protecting communities against vaccine-preventable diseases.

FURTHER READING

"Assessing the State of Vaccine Confidence in the United States: Recommendations from the National Vaccine Advisory Committee." 2015. *Public Health Reports* 130 (6): 573–95. https://doi.org/10.1177/0033354 91513000606.

National Public Health Information Coalition. 2021. "Rebuilding Trust in Public Health." https://www.nphic.org/cvirus-ate-commseries.

National Science Foundation (NSF). 2021. "NSF invests $21 Million to Tackle 2 Complex Societal Challenges: The Networked Blue Economy, and Trust and Authenticity in Communication Systems." https://www.nsf.gov/news/special_reports/announcements/092221.jsp.

National Vaccine Program Office. 2017. *The Vaccine Confidence Meeting.* https://www.hhs.gov/sites/default/files/2017-vaccine-confidence-meeting-report.pdf.

U.S. Department of Health and Human Services (HHS). 2021. *Confronting Health Misinformation: The U.S. Surgeon General's Advisory on Building a Healthy Information Environment.* https://www.hhs.gov/sites/default/files/surgeon-general-misinformation-advisory.pdf.

U.S. Department of Health and Human Services (HHS). n.d. "Featured Priorities: Vaccine Confidence." Accessed October 18, 2021. https://www.hhs.gov/vaccines/featured-priorities/vaccine-confidence/index.html.

World Health Organization (WHO). n.d. "About Vaccine Safety Net." Accessed October 14, 2021. https://vaccinesafetynet.org/vsn/vaccine-safety-net.

World Health Organization (WHO). n.d. "Early AI-Supported Response with Social Listening." Accessed October 14, 2021. https://www.who-ears.com.

Index